HEALTHY Hair REHAB NOW

HEALTHY Hair REHAB NOW

3 Steps to Fabulous Healthy Hair

By **Hair-ologist** Jacqueline Tarrant

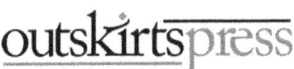

outskirts press

DENVER, COLORADO

This book is lovingly dedicated
to the most important people in my life:

*My wonderful mother Corene Tarrant who did not give me life,
but gave me an amazing life.

*My sister Judy, whose dedication to family is second to none—
Thanks for always having my back.

*My fiancé Courtney who believes in me and
supports my dreams through thick and thin.

My clients: I dedicate this labor of love to you and hope it will help
in some small way to make your hair experience better.

Table of Contents

Introduction: Meet the Hair Expert Who Has Given Hair Advice to Millions —

As a third-generation beauty professional, my life's passion has been the pursuit of everything hair. Following my great-aunt and my mother, now it's my turn to carry on the pursuit of healthy, stylish hair. Having been surrounded by hair care my entire life, and having literally been raised in mother's salon, it feels like second nature to crave everything hair. No, really — the crib was in the corner and combs, brushes, and clips were my toys of choice. I was mixing a highlighting solution to bleach my doll's hair at the age of three, when my mother discovered my busy hands at work. She nearly had a fit, exclaiming, "I knew you were too quiet, you had to be into something." She later laughed but could not dampen my determination to digest every cut, color, curl, and wave I saw. I would fall asleep leaning on her as she worked, not wanting to miss anything. Every day I remember her busily laughing, talking, and making ladies look fabulous one by one until finally it was time to go home. I loved salon life so much that I would cry to go with her rather than stay home, even on weekends. Everyone said I was spoiled, always stuck under my mom, but I loved to watch her work magic, because one day it would be my turn — and then one day it was.

I started off as a shampoo assistant and worked my way up to my own chair. Working in the salon after school every day was actually fun for me and I continued, even through college. Momma encouraged me to go to college and to keep my options open. I had two parents who stressed education as the key to success. Because of that, I have always had a hunger to learn. It was great having my own clients and making my own money. I had completed my apprentice program in the salon, but still wanted to be sure I could pass the State Board of Cosmetology test. To be sure of my success, while still in college, I enrolled in beauty school at night and found that I knew more than I thought. In many instances, I knew more than my teachers. Armed with that confidence, I aced my State Board test. When I got my first job out of college, I still came into the salon after work because my clients were important to me. After working at unfulfilling jobs, I eventually went into the salon full time to start my career and loved every minute of it. Before long, I had a booming clientele. I soon became a platform artist for SoftSheen Products and had the excitement of world travel, educating other beauty professionals and consumers about the features and benefits of popular brands like Mizani and Optimum, to name a few.

In 1999, L'Oréal purchased Soft Sheen Products, and in 2000, I was offered the opportunity to relocate to Chicago, IL from Baltimore, MD to work under the title of Product Development Specialist. This really took my career in beauty to the next level. I left my salon and moved into a corporate environment. A salon space was set up for me to test products and work closely with the chemist and brand marketers to develop products that could be purchased from beauty store shelves. In 2001, L'Oréal acquired Carson's Product which added Dark & Lovely, Let's Jam, and Magic Shave to the portfolio, to name a few. The horizons were broadening and it was an amazing experience working with such a diverse portfolio of brands.

The long and short of it is, I traveled the world promoting and educating about the brands, and worked with some amazing people to continue to create new and innovative brands. I became director of education and was spokesperson for SoftSheen-Carson with magazines like *The Wall Street Journal*, *Seventeen,* and *Essence.* The TV appearances on *Good Morning America*, Fox, NBC, ABC and CBS were absolutely amazing. Somehow I kept feeling as if I should be doing more.

I noticed that there is an entire community of women suffering from hair damage, hair breakage, thinning, and hair loss issues. Unfortunately, these same women are not connecting with any understanding about the root cause of their problems. These women do not know the steps to avoid hair loss issues. I studied with the best to learn more about hair loss. My passion became focused on creating a place where individuals could come and get an easy understanding of the contributing factors to hair damage and loss. Understanding the cause and effect is priceless. Not just treatment, but more importantly prevention through education is the key to success.

Around the same time of my epiphany, my mother began to experience some health challenges associated with the aging process. I wanted to have a bit more freedom and flexibility to share the challenge of caring for her. So the obvious thing was to resign and pursue the next phase of my life. With that act of faith, I founded the Hair Trauma Center in downtown Chicago, IL. I have been able to help numerous women and men to understand and treat their hair problems. Most people don't realize that there are at least seven causes of hair loss and numerous causes of hair breakage. There are always steps one can take to avoid, prevent, overcome, or slow down a process of hair breakage and loss. My daily purpose is to educate, enlighten, and empower women and men with the knowledge of these causes and the steps to prevent hair loss and breakage.

The purpose of this book is to share much of this information with you, with the hope that you or someone you know can have one less bad hair day. Yes, the impact of a perception of a bad hair day or the idea of bad hair can have a devastating impact on an individual. You'll read more about that later — but first things first: let's learn a little about your hair.

1

Getting to the Root of the Problem:

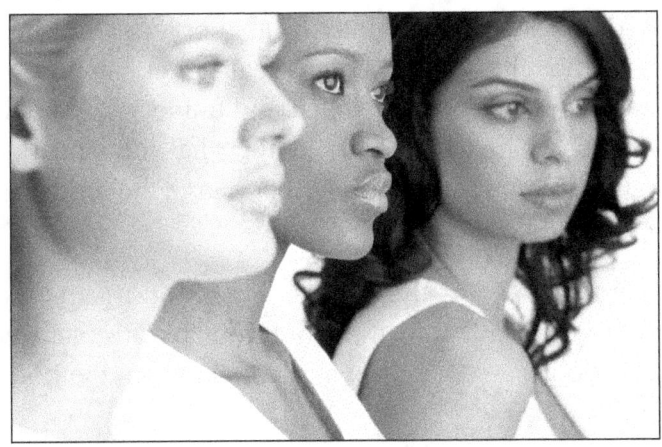

Hair damage, hair breakage, or hair loss strikes a sense of fear and frustration into anyone suffering through it. When faced with strand fallout you may think you're the only one, but one out of three people will experience noticeable hair loss. At some point in time almost every woman has been concerned with hair breakage or loss. These concerns are not unique to any culture or group but stretch across race, culture, and hair type and texture. Women with highly textured and fine hair may find their hair to be more fragile and therefore may have more even challenges with care and maintenance.

The problem of dry and brittle hair is one of the most common complaints that I hear through my hair advice columns and when conducting client consultations. This problem often leads to breakage and is second only to the complaint of fragile and thinning hair. Though dry, fragile, or thinning hair is the noticeable and obvious problem, it is usually a symptom or side effect of a bigger problem. The most common response may lead one to reach for the moisturizer or the protein conditioner. Most of us are under the assumption that slathering the area with a creamy conditioner is the cure. I would like to challenge you to look at the big picture and consider your hair as a barometer of the body's balance and well-being. It is important to ask the right questions. Yes, over the years you may have pulled it, fried it, dyed it, permed it, braided it, abandoned it, and abused it. Though these merciless acts may have caused collateral damage, at the most basic level, your hair's sheen and fullness may not be about how much you've abused it. Truly healthy hair depends largely on your changing hormones, the pills you pop, and the foods and beverages you eat or don't eat.

Your hair is nourished directly through your bloodstream, so anything that gets into your body and therefore your bloodstream will have an impact on your hair. Likewise, any imbalance in the body will be noticeable in the hair.

My goal is to help you begin to probe deeper when hair issues arise. Don't overlook the obvious. Is it an external issue (outside of the body, the hair we can touch) caused from pulling hair too tight, over processing relaxers, overdoing hair color, or too much heat? Or is it an internal issue (inside your body) from a lack of proper nutrition, hormone imbalance, dehydration, the side effect of medication, declining health condition, genetics, or a combination of factors?

In the following pages we will probe into all of the above, and I hope you will allow me this opportunity to share a different approach to your hair issues in a new and more comprehensive way.

From this day forward, look beyond the surface of the problem: probe a little deeper. Cross check your hair facts with your health facts to better determine the root of your hair issues.

Three Steps to Success

Step 1: Probe

Investigate — look beyond the surface — discover:

In order to fully understand your hair issues, you will need to look beyond the surface. Far too often we reach for the conditioner of choice to correct hair trauma. Hair breakage, hair thinning, shedding, and loss can be a complicated scenario. Conditioner cannot cure all of your hair ills. Get to the source of the problem.

Is hair breaking because of chemical damage from hair color or perms, or is there a deeper issue, perhaps an internal health issue driving the hair loss process? A consultation with a professional should reveal the possible source through a series of questions and tests. As you continue to read, you can begin your probe to get to the root of any hair issues you may be experiencing. At some point you will discover the next step to provide your hair with the rehab it requires to get to the fabulous hair you would love to have.

Step 2: Prescribe

A plan of care — a customized plan of action just for you and your unique hair issues:

Once your problem has been revealed, you should have a course of action recommended to get an improved result. Perhaps it will be as simple as reducing the strength of the relaxer you're currently using. On the other hand, you may have a scalp fungus that is damaging your hair follicles, and this is the reason your hair is falling out. In this instance, your dermatologist can prescribe medication and scalp creams to kill bacteria and heal the scalp. A healthy scalp will promote healthy hair growth. Regardless of the diagnosis, once you have been provided with a solution, it becomes necessary for you to follow the advice given to get a positive result.

Step 3: Persist

To continue steadfastly or firmly — to maintain a course of action with the objective of success and long-term maintenance:

Again, follow the treatment plan given and be consistent; this is the only way you will get the fabulous result you desire.

The Real Purpose of Hair:

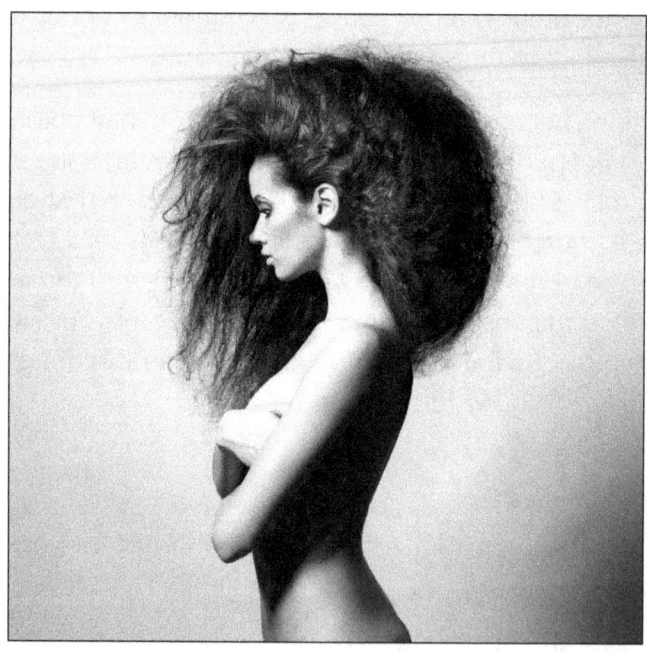

Today, many view hair as an accessory, but in ancient times when we lived in the elements, under trees, or in caves, hair helped to keep us warm. Our hair was our coat and helped to protect parts of our body from the elements.

Believe it or not, each of us starts out with an average of 100,000 – 150,000 strands of hair on the head. Hair serves multiple purposes.

The original purpose was to keep the warmth in and to protect us from overexposure to the sun. Hair provides natural insulation. The majority of our body heat escapes through the head (an important part of temperature regulation). Hair provides insulation when the body temperature begins to drop.

Even Before Birth, Hair Is Present:

By week 22, a developing fetus has all of its hair follicles formed. At this stage of life there are about 5 million hair follicles on the body. The head has a total of one million, with one hundred thousand of those follicles residing on the scalp. This is the largest number of hair follicles a human will ever have, since we do not generate new hair follicles anytime during the course of our lives. Most people will notice that the density of scalp hair is reduced as they grow from childhood to adulthood. The reason: our scalps expand as we grow.

How does hair grow?

Hair has two distinct structures: first, the follicle itself, which resides in the skin; and second, the shaft, which is visible above the scalp.

The hair follicle is a tunnel-like segment of the skin's epidermis that extends down into the dermis. The structure contains several layers that all have separate functions. At the base of the follicle is the papilla, which contains capillaries, or tiny blood vessels that nourish the cells. The living part of the hair is the very bottom part surrounding the papilla, called the bulb. The cells of the bulb divide every 23 to 72 hours, faster than any other cell in the body.

Two sheaths, an inner and outer sheath, surround the follicle. These structures protect and form the growing hair shaft. The inner sheath follows the hair shaft and ends below the opening of a sebaceous (oil) gland and sometimes an apocrine (scent) gland. The outer sheath continues all the way up to the gland. A muscle called an erector pili muscle attaches below the gland to a fibrous layer around the outer sheath. When this muscle contracts, it causes the hair to stand up, which also causes the sebaceous gland to secrete oil.

The sebaceous gland is vital because it produces sebum, or natural oil lubricant, which conditions the hair and skin. During puberty our body produces more sebum, but as we age we begin to make less sebum. Women have far less sebum production than men do as they age.

To simplify all of that biology, the follicles (which will be discussed often in the following pages) are tiny hair growing factories under the scalp. The follicles are nourished mainly by the protein in your daily diet, and by carbohydrates such as whole grains (they provide energy); essential fatty acids from fish, nuts and soy (they hydrate the follicle); vitamins B6, B12, and Biotin found in eggs, bananas, salmon, and spinach (they help strengthen your hair's outer layer, called the cuticle; this is the area you can touch). Iron is also essential to the turnover and replenishment of the hair strand. Keep in mind that this is a process. It takes 90 days for a cell to rejuvenate. If you begin eating for hair health today and remain consistent, it will be reflected in approximately 12 weeks, or 3 months. Hair grows at about one-quarter to one-half inch per month. If your hair is shoulder length, your longest strands are about 2 years old. If you start adding healthy portions of fatty acids and B12 right now, your hair should begin to look better in 3 to 6 months, so *Bon Appétit!*

2 | The Power of Hair

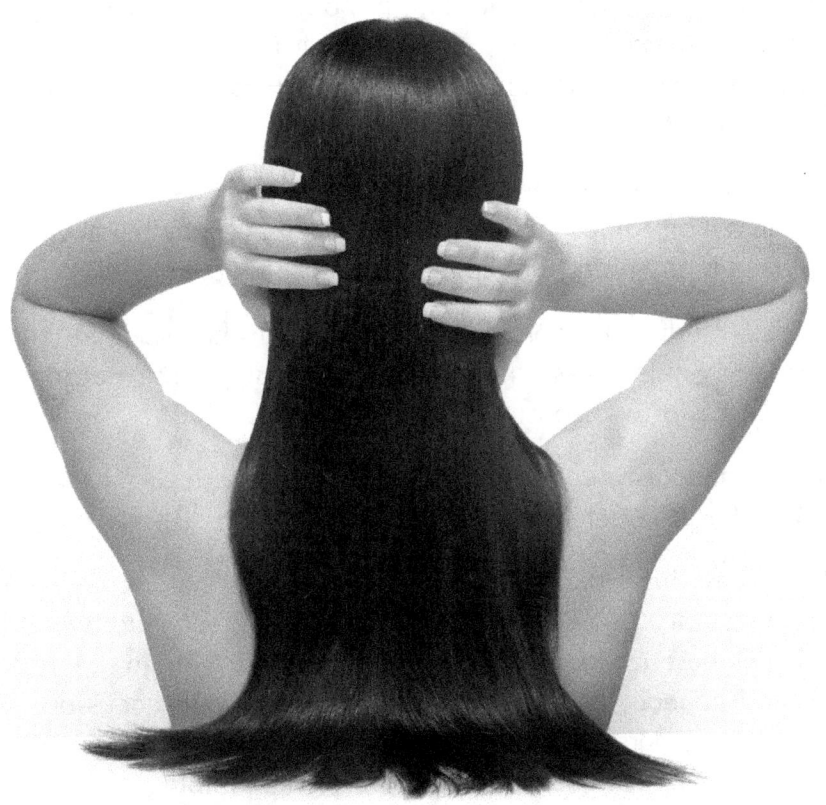

Throughout history people have been obsessed with their hair. Many cultures have equated luxurious locks with youth, virility, stamina, strength, beauty, and sensuality. For as long as records have been kept, hair on the head has been considered a sexual object. For thousands of years, its texture, styling, length, color, and other attributes have been among the charismatic standards of adornment in almost every civilization.

Do you know why Julius Cesar wore a wreath of leaves? It was to hide his hair loss, a receded forehead and bare-scalp crown. In some cultures, women, prisoners, and soldiers are forced to hide their hair or shave it to symbolize a lack of individuality or sexuality. Look at what happens to the heads of recruits newly entered into the armed forces. Their heads are clean-shaven, both to take away dignity and to separate them from being distinct entities unto themselves. Some might say removing head hair makes someone a non-person with no distinct identity.

Hair connotes power and has symbolized sturdiness for men. When Delilah cut off Sampson's hair, he lost the great strength, which characterized him. As a result, the Philistines captured him.

American Indian warriors believed that when they scalped the enemy, they would possess his strength and courage. The warrior with the most scalps was considered the most powerful.

Documented research into hair loss and hair growth goes back 6,000 years to Egypt's Ancient Kingdom.

How many times have you heard the phrase, "hair is a woman's crowning glory"? In evolution, early men looked for mates with long and thick hair because it was an indication of a woman's reproductive and general health. Many feel that hair is an accessory and don't fully understand the power of hair until they experience hair issues such as hair breakage, damage, hair thinning or hair loss. For many the hair experience is very powerful, and should never be dismissed as trivial. The truth is that men and women tie a lot of self-esteem to their hair.

At some point, everyone has experienced what has become popularly known as a "bad hair day." In many cases, the phrase is used to indicate the overall experience of an unpleasant day. For anyone who has ever suffered from frizzy locks, limp locks, or cowlicks, it will come as no surprise to hear that researchers have now demonstrated that bad hair days may actually have a negative impact on self-esteem. Bad hair may not only be a style challenge, it may also be harmful to your mental health.

In a study commissioned by *Physique*, researchers at Yale University found that "bad hair days" impact self-esteem by increasing levels of self-doubt and personal criticism. "Interestingly, both women and men are negatively affected by the phenomenon of bad hair days," says Dr. Marianne LaFrance, Professor of Psychology and Professor of Women's and Gender Studies at Yale University. "Even more fascinating is our finding that individuals perceive their capabilities to be significantly lower than others when experiencing bad hair."

Participants in the study included both men and women of diverse ethnicity from varied cultural backgrounds. Researchers were particularly interested in how bad hair days affected individuals on measures of self-esteem, social insecurity, and feelings of personal value. One of the most interesting findings of the study was that bad hair days had a dramatic impact on performance and self-esteem. The experience of a bad hair day caused study participants to feel less smart and less capable at performing tasks in which they were normally competent. Most surprisingly, this effect was highest among men.

The study also showed a dramatic increase in social insecurity among those suffering from a bad hair day. The reason for this is fairly simple. When we are anxious about an aspect of our appearance, we tend to believe that others are also noticing our perceived imperfections. In many cases, other people notice such things far less than we imagine. In the Yale study, women reported experiencing more feelings of shame and embarrassment while men reported lowered confidence and increased nervousness. In addition to this social anxiety about appearance, study participants began making other negative comments about themselves. Researchers concluded that "bad hair days" could lead to other feelings of self-criticism that go far beyond appearance.

Women Speak:

Findings from a new national telephone poll of 1031 women suggest that bad hair days are bad news days for almost half the female population. Lisa Lee Freeman, editor in chief of *Shop Smart*, conducted the poll. The magazine is published by *Consumer Reports*. "Hair is a big thing for women, and if it's not behaving, it can be a bit traumatizing because you still have to walk out of the house and be seen in public."

The poll showed that 44 percent of women say their mood has been affected by a bad hair day. A fourth (26 percent) has cried after getting a haircut and a third have regretted a style change.

Women's biggest gripes about their hair:

- too thin or fine
- color
- too curly or frizzy
- too dry or damaged
- too thick
- too much time to style
- too straight
- unmanageable
- graying
- falling out

The Price of Pretty:

According to a survey conducted by Tresemme, the average woman spends a staggering $50,000 on her hair over her lifetime. If you wear extensions in your hair you can double, triple, or quadruple that amount based on the cost of the hair and the stylist.

An Investment of Time:

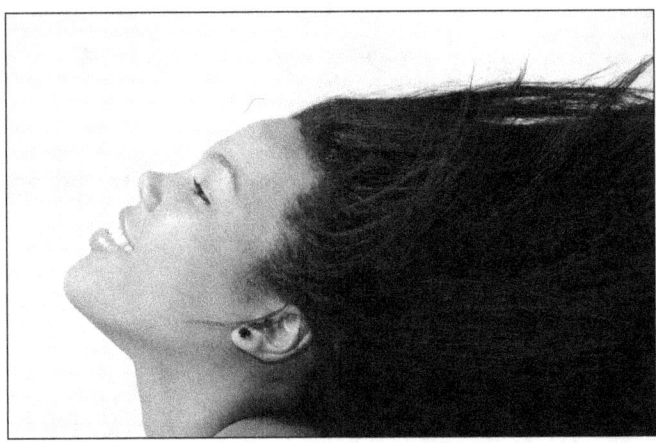

A beauty survey commissioned by the British beauty brand Nephria found women spend almost three years of their life getting ready to leave the house, according to *Marie Claire* magazine. According to the study, women spend an average of one hour and 53 minutes a week shampooing, blow drying, and styling our hair. That may not sound like a lot, but by the time a woman reaches the age of 65, she will have spent more than seven months of her life on her hair! For women with highly textured hair that number could double or even triple. Who knew?

Know Your Hair:

It's your hair — how well do you know it?

- Do you know the present condition of your hair?
- Do you know the type and texture of your hair?
- Do you know how many strands to expect in your daily hair shed routine?
- Do you know the difference between shedding and breakage?
- Do you know your hair's genetic pre-disposition for thinning?

You may ask why you should know these Personal Hair Facts (PHF). Your PHF hold the key to your hair's future, and most importantly, knowing your PHF can help you maximize your hair's style, health, and beauty. Knowing can bring you peace of mind.

Personal Hair Facts You Should Know:

Know the condition of your hair — Is your hair damaged?

How do you identify damaged hair?
- Roughened cuticle layer
- Porous, tends to split
- Very difficult to comb
- Looks dull, feels like straw
- No strength or vitality
- Conditions vary from roots to ends
- Damaged hair has a rough texture and low elasticity. Healthy hair can stretch and return to its original shape without breaking.
- Dry brittle hair breaks easily and cannot hold a curl from thermal styling or permanent waving. It appears frayed and rough.
- Damaged hair is overly porous and dries quickly.

Chemically Damaged Hair:
The overuse of chemicals such as permanent hair color and bleaching lighteners are the fastest way to damage hair. Chemically damaged hair feels brittle and often looks like straw.

Thermal Damaged Hair:
The daily use of blow dryers, hot rollers, curling irons, flat irons, and straighteners can affect hair health. A hot tool can burn and singe hair. If the thermal tool is too hot it will create a strong odor and even singe the hair strands. This is causing damage to the hair. The glue-like and spring-like proteins in your hair shift every time you heat the hair with thermal tools. It is this action that allows the hair to take on the shape of the hot roller, curling iron, or flat iron.

Here's a tip — Test before you touch:

Test your hot tool on a white tissue or paper towel. If the paper turns brown, then cool down your iron until it does not singe the paper. If it will burn the paper, it will definitely burn your hair.

Prescription Drug Effects:

Medications for rheumatoid arthritis can cause brittle hair and hair loss. Chemotherapy for cancer causes the hair to fall out. The hair sometimes grows back a different color and texture. Bipolar medications, such as lithium, can also damage the hair. (In Chapter 7 you will find a list of medications that have a side effect of hair loss).

Damage from the Environment:

UV rays from the sun can cause dryness to the hair and fade hair color. Well water can make hair resistant to chemical services. Minerals from hard water can also strip the hair and give it a brittle appearance.

Know your *Hair Texture:*

Texture is the size of your hair strand:

- Is your hair fine, or a narrow/slender-sized strand?
- Is your hair medium?
- Is your hair coarse?

Know your *Hair Type:*

- Is your hair straight?
- Is your hair wavy?
- Is your hair curly, excessively curly or kinky?

This information is important when choosing shampoos, conditioners, or chemical products like chemical straightener, permanent wave, or heat setting on flat iron or other hot tools.

Know your **Hair Density** (the number of hair strands per square inch)

- Is your hair thick, moderate, or thin?

This information is very important when deciding how much product you're going to use and how much time it may take to apply the product. A perfect example is if you are planning to color really thick hair at home. Always follow the manufacturer's instructions regarding instructions for use, but make sure how much product you will need. You may need to buy more than one box of color. If your hair is really long and thick, you may need to buy up to three or more boxes of color. I promise you that it will not be fun to start applying hair color and run out of color before you're finished.

3 | Un-break My Hair!

Is Your Hair Breaking or Shedding?

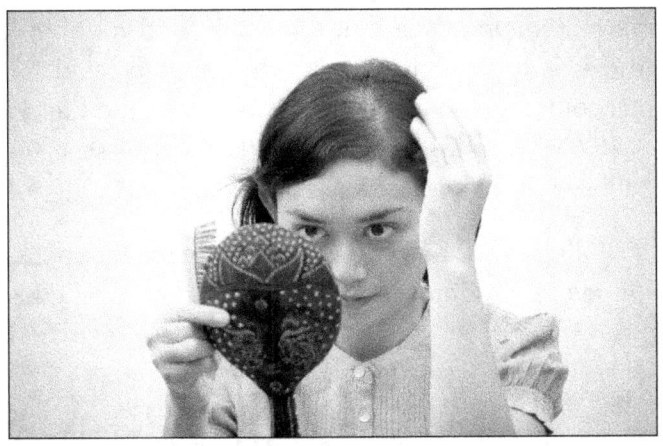

Shedding is natural. Hair strands that are shed will be the full length of the strand and will have a small white bulb attached at the root. Shed strands will usually result from a natural **internal function** or bodily malfunction.

Breakage is unnatural. Breakage may be in short or medium-length pieces. A broken strand is an external result of a weakened strand. A weakened strand may break easily with external manipulation, such as combing, brushing, or styling. The breakage may be the result of chemical over processing from hair straighteners, curly perms, permanent hair color, hair bleach, highlights, or weakening of the strand from extreme heat styling. All of these chemical applications and techniques can result in an excessive loss of protein and moisture, leaving hair fragile to the touch and easily broken.

How Much Is Too Much Hair to Lose in a Day?

In the daily course of our lives, we lose hair through everyday actions such as shampooing, combing, and brushing. Many people find this is cause for concern as they do not understand the process of hair growth and don't know when or if they should worry about their hair falling out.

Here is some help in understanding what hair shed you should expect, and how much is too much. The average human head has around 100,000 hair follicles. On average, blondes have the highest density of hair at 140,000 hair follicles; redheads the lowest at 90,000 follicles; and those with dark hair have on average 110,000 follicles.

Human hair follicles are perhaps the only organs that actually grow in a specific cycle. During the growth cycle, our hair goes through three stages:

1. **Anagen**: This is the growing stage of human hair. It lasts anywhere from 2 to 5 years and as much as 85-90 percent of our hair is usually in the growing phase. Some people cannot grow the hair past shoulder length. Others can grow their hair down to their ankles. The length of your anagen cycle helps determine the length to which you can grow your hair.

2. **Catagen**: After the anagen phase, our hair enters into the catagen phase, which is a small regression phase. It is kind of a transition stage between the anagen and telogen phases. This phase lasts around 2-3 weeks and about 1 percent of hair is in this phase at any given time.

3. **Telogen**: This is the last and resting phase of human hair. At

any given time, 10-15 percent of hair is in this phase, which can last around 3-4 months. In this phase the hair is just sitting on your body and basically waiting to fall out.

It is normal to lose hair through our daily hair care, but what is "normal" varies from person to person, and therefore so does what is "excessive." The denser your hair and the shorter your anagen cycle, the more hair you will naturally lose per day. For example, suppose your hair is blond and your average anagen + catagen + telogen cycle lasts 3 years. That means every year about 47,000 hairs are replaced. That is equivalent to losing an average of 127 hairs per day normally. Suppose you are a redhead and your anagen + catagen + telogen cycle lasts 5 years. That would mean that on average you lose 90,000 per year, or about 50 hairs per day. While losing 130 hairs a day regularly may be normal for one person, it could be excessive for another.

Obviously, there is no way to actually count how many strands of hair you lose every day. Your daily hair care routine may promote hair breakage, but probably won't be the cause of excessive hair loss. If you are experiencing excessive hair loss, it will be because of some internal underlying causes such as genetics, hormonal imbalance, medications, etc.

We'll go into more details about excessive hair shedding in a later chapter. You don't want to miss it!

What Causes Breakage?

We have established that a certain amount of shedding is normal. Breakage, on the other hand, is not natural and is an indication of an imbalance of important forces within the hair strand. When the normal balance of protein and moisture for your hair is not maintained, the external hair shaft may break off. Broken hairs do not fall naturally from the head, but are typically a sign of mishandling or abuse. In the stages before a hair strand ultimately breaks, it experiences cuticle loss, which weakens the hair shaft. Eventually, the fibers begin to split or unravel and ultimately there is breakage.

So, what causes breakage? Hair can be weakened and damaged by anything from rough handling and sun exposure to coloring and straightening chemicals. Breakage is also more common with a hair strand's age; older hairs, usually nearest the ends, have the greatest tendency to break due to normal wear and tear. When breakage isn't a response to physical manipulation and abuse, it is most often triggered by the lack of moisture in the hair strand. Other types of breakage may be caused by the over-structuring of the hair strand with protein treatments done in excess.

No Rough Stuff, Please

Rough physical handling of the hair can damage the hair. Aggressive brushing, combing of tangled hair, and other grooming techniques can put a lot of physical stress on the hair strand and can cause the strand to break. This is known as friction and is one of the top causes of hair breakage.

Hair is at its weakest point when it is wet, so handle with extreme caution and care. To avoid this type of breakage, gently towel blot wet hair first, then lightly apply a leave-in detangling conditioner to minimize tangles and snarls. Use a wide-tooth comb with smooth tips, not sharp or broken teeth. Begin combing one section at a time, gently combing from the ends to the root.

The excessive use of extremely hot hair dryers can cause a lot of damage. When you shampoo your hair, some water gets under the cuticle and into the cortex. If you attempt to dry your soaking wet hair with a high heat, you heat up the water. This makes the water expand inside the hair and this literally pushes outward to leave spaces in the hair fiber. In severe cases the hair develops little bubbles inside, a condition appropriately called "bubble hair." These bubbles make the hair much weaker and likely to break off.

Again, hair is at its weakest point when it is wet, so lightly towel blot excess water from the hair. Take controlled sections, and use warm to hot air over and around hair, directing hair in the desired styling direction.

Hair comes in a variety of textures from fine to coarse. Hair can suffer a range of damage, from fraying split ends to damage caused by straightening hair with chemical agents or hair irons. There can also be hair damage due to heat from blow dryers or curling irons, or hair coloring problems.

Heat

Whether your hair is chemically processed or natural, too much heat can hurt it. This pertains to daily heat abuse through the use of flat irons, curling irons, or pressing combs. It also applies to high temperatures used even once. Hair can and *will* burn if extremely hot tools are used on it. Unfortunately, some women have found this out the hard way. When temperatures are too high, the spring-like and glue-like proteins are permanently shifted to a position of weakness in the cortex inner layer. An extreme loss of moisture and protein render the hair weak, and breakage is inevitable.

Is Hair Loss in Your Genes?

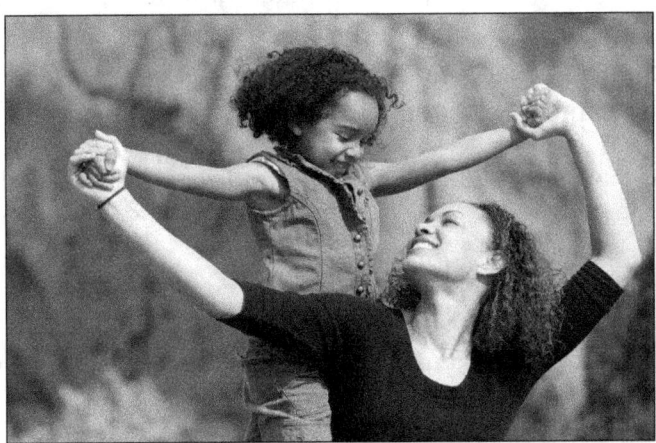

In many instances, thinning hair is more a result of your genetic make-up than any other reason. You may have heard the myth about wearing hats or shampooing too often. The most common cause of hair loss is genetic in nature and is clinically known as Androgenetic Alopecia.

Chances are your scalp's fate has been predetermined in the womb. The hair follicles are genetically programmed, much like all of your other body parts. Included in this program is the time and extent of the baldness you will incur in your entire lifetime. Hair thinning occurs when specific hormones affect those hair follicles which carry an innate susceptibility to their effects. The human body can manufacture male hormones. This function disregards gender factors, and is applicable to women as well. The two hormones usually produced are dihydrotestosterone (DHT), and testosterone. On the other hand, the hair follicles and skin pores are abundant in an enzyme known as 5-alpha-reductase; this substance can convert testosterone into dihydrotestosterone (DHT) through the help of the bloodstream. An overabundance of this single hormone, DHT, is known as the primary cause of male-pattern baldness. Some people have an inborn vulnerability to baldness at the top of their heads. During maturity or middle age, this area is specifically targeted by DHT by binding with the receptors of the susceptible follicles, causing the latter to eventually weaken. Now the normal growth cycle of a hair follicle is three to eight years; at the end of this process, the shaft and strand are separated from the hair follicle, in place of a new strand. With hair thinning, the growth cycles gets progressively shorter in time, and the hair strand that comes out of the follicle becomes ever thinner in volume and thickness. This process is known as miniaturization.

This cycle successively takes on a gradual severity, and will eventually lead to baldness in most of the people who experience it.

Is Hair Loss the Same for Men and Women?

The difference between Female Pattern Balding (FPB) and Male Pattern Balding (MPB) is primarily in the type of pattern that emerges as hair loss progresses. Though both men and women can have both MPB and/or FPB, it is usually men who have MPB and women who have FPB. MPB is characterized by a receding hairline and temples and the formation of a bald spot at the crown of the scalp. As MPB progresses, the bald spot becomes larger and the hair line moves higher and higher until the hair at the top or vertex of the scalp is completely gone. In even the most severe cases of MPB hair remains intact at the sides and at the back of the head. In FPB, there is essentially an overall thinning out of the hair on top of the head while the hair line remains intact, except in the most severe cases. Usually in FPB, one still has enough hair that it gives coverage to the scalp (i.e. no slick bald spots typically form), however if you part the hair you'll notice a bigger gap at the part.

The relationship we have with our hair is the ultimate in love/hate relationships for many of us. You may blame those bad hair days on harsh winter weather, humidity, or styling products gone wrong. Have you considered that the condition of your hair may reflect the condition of your health? You probably won't have healthy hair if you don't have a healthy body. If you're dealing with hair that's dull, dry, frizzy, flaky, or falling out, it's worth a closer look to make sure it's not due to something bigger than just using the wrong shampoo. From genetics to your current nutritional state, learning to read your hair can tell you a lot about your overall health.

Hair follicles must receive a steady flow of nutrients in order to remain healthy. The follicles receive their nutrients through the blood supply. If circulation is poor, follicles will become malnourished; the root will suffer, causing the hair not to grow to its full potential. The increased blood supply helps to nourish and energize the follicles.

Additional Causes of Hair Breakage and Hair Loss:

- Protein Deficiency (often associated with recent significant weight loss)
- Iron Deficiency
- Thyroid Disease
- Anemia
- Severe Mental Stress
- Auto Immune Disease
- Prescription Drug Side Effects
- Hormonal Imbalance
- Hair Loss After Pregnancy

- Aging Hair and Menopause
- Vitamin and Nutrient Deficiency
- Chemical and Heat Abuse
- Physical Hair Shaft Trauma (Traction Alopecia)

Severe Mental Stress, often defined as anxiety and worry, may affect your body and mind, as you try to deal with your emotional issues. When the body and health are negatively affected (i.e., trauma, pregnancy, emotional stress, major illness) your hair no longer has priority for your health maintenance. It's as if your body is saying, *"I've got bigger problems to worry about, I don't need to worry about hair growth right now."*

Your body's built-in self-healing "process" considers your other problems so important that it concentrates on the problems and ignores your hair. A sudden or stressful event can cause the hair follicles to prematurely stop growing and enter into a resting phase. This process, known as telogen effluvium, occurs when more hairs go into a "resting phase" and are shed. The one thing that everyone must understand about their hair is that it serves no vital function for our health. Without it, we can live and function normally. Centuries ago, the hair on the heads of our early ancestors kept their heads warm and reduced heat loss. However, for the most part, this is no longer necessary in today's modern society.

Although women don't have nearly as much testosterone as men, when women undergo intense stress, the adrenal glands become overworked due to an increased need for the "stress hormone" known as cortisol. This causes the body to produce more adrenaline and testosterone, and DHT, a stronger variant of testosterone. The increased production of these hormones can sometimes cause the hair to fall out due to the resulting hormonal imbalance.

Telogen effluvium is characterized by sudden diffuse hair loss caused by an interruption in the normal hair growth cycle. This interruption is often the result of trauma, such as chemotherapy, childbirth, major surgery, severe stress, or severe chronic illness. This trauma causes large numbers of hair follicles to enter a stage of telogen, or rest, simultaneously.

The telogen phase can last 6 to 12 weeks (and much longer if left untreated) and seems to affect women much more than men. Stress factors that can lead to temporary hair loss:

- Death of family member, friend, or spouse
- Accident
- Intense work-related stress
- Financial problems
- Divorce
- Major illness or surgery
- Childbirth

The good news is that stress-related hair loss (telogen effluvium) is temporary. In fact, due to the nature of the hair growth cycle, by the time your hair starts to shed heavily, your stress-related problem might have already been resolved.

Tips for handling stress:

- *Exercising* for just 20 minutes a day can produce enough endorphins to reduce stress levels.

- **Write in a journal,** capturing and releasing your thoughts and feelings every day. Surprisingly, this can help in expressing the frustrations you are keeping inside. The writing process can also help you to work through your emotions and find a resolution you can embrace. Be patient with yourself and don't be afraid to ask for help.

- **Get a massage.** Massage therapy can relax muscles, ease muscle spasms, increase blood flow to skin and muscles, and relieve mental and emotional stress.

4

Weaves, Braids, and Other Tight Situations

Weaves, Braids, and Extensions — if it's Too Tight, it's Not Right!

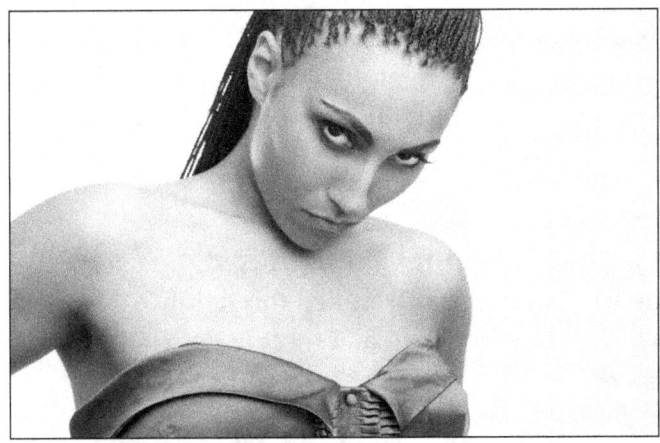

With traction alopecia, the cause may involve things like tight braids, pulling the hair into a tight ponytail, cornrow hairstyles, and anything else that pulls on the roots of the hair. Sometimes the follicles are damaged to the extent that they stop growing, resulting in permanent hair loss.

The styles themselves are not the problem — it's only when they are done incorrectly, meaning too tight; that's when the problem rears its ugly head. As a beauty professional, I am not anti-weave, anti-braids, or anti-ponytail. In fact, at some point I've worn them all. I am, however, against performing a service improperly, and causing long-term damage to an unknowing individual.

I hear this all the time during consultations: "I thought the weave/ braids would help, by giving my hair a rest." It is important to know that if hair is weak, fragile, or thinning the tension, tightness, and stress of a weave or braids will probably be too much. I cannot stress this enough: these styles when done too tight and on fragile hair can be the trigger for hair loss, which could end up being permanent.

Traction Alopecia

Traction alopecia is caused by damage done to the hair follicle by continual pulling and tight tension for very long periods. This type of hair loss has been on the rise and is one of the fastest growing areas in dermatology, as people continue to damage their hair. It occurs in people who wear tight braids and dreadlocks that lead to pulling, tension, and breaking of hair.

Traction Alopecia Happens in 3 Steps:

1. The **hair is consistently pulled too tightly** causing hair strands to loosen from the follicular roots (where hair starts the growth process).

2. Trauma causes **follicular inflammation** (or small itchy bumps). The bumps are the outward appearance of the presence of inflammatory cells within the wall of the hair follicle.

3. Atrophy **(shrinkage) of the follicle**. With persistent tightly pulled hair, the damaged follicles will progressively decrease in size and no longer produce the typical long and coarse hair. Instead, thinner, weaker, more fragile fine, short hair is generated, and eventually it will not produce hair at all. The follicle will shut down; the scalp pore will close and become a smooth surface.

African-American women seem to be affected more than men who braid their hair or have dreadlocks. Traction alopecia occurs more commonly in teenagers and young adults more than it does in older people, unless they also damage their hair in the same ways. In most cases, people do not realize that it is damaging to hair as well as the hair follicles.

The only way to stop the damaging effect is to catch it early enough and stop the damaging process. Hairstyles that put tension on the hair follicles have to change for the best results. African-American women are vulnerable to traction alopecia. Hair stylists specializing in braids and chemical processing should warn about traction alopecia and advise customers on the risks.

Many products suggest that conditioning the hair follicles and cleansing the scalp will revitalize damaged hair from traction alopecia. This is not always the case; hair loss sustained by constant abuse remains damaged for life. The early detection of this form of alopecia might be able to be corrected, but prolonged abuse without proper care can be irreversible.

In the early stages of hair loss, you may also need to discontinue all forms of styling your hair. The hair follicles need to rejuvenate and grow hair as if you were starting out as a baby. With any kind of hair damage, you must determine how bad it is, as well as how much of the head and hair was damaged by this process. A proper scalp analysis by a certified professional can provide a snapshot of your hair's condition.

Once you have determined these facts, a restoration specialist can prescribe treatment as well as recommend alternatives. The best treatment is to stop causing tension to the hair follicles — now. The hair needs to grow out and remain loose in order to grow properly. Society does not warn about improper hair care, but is quick to provide some questionable remedies to the problem. Do not be fooled into thinking, as many are, that your hair grows back after years of abuse. This is not going to happen. If you are lucky enough to learn early, you will save thousands of dollars by growing healthy hair.

If you choose to wear tight hairstyles, you will want to undo the styles weekly in order to prevent traction alopecia from becoming a problem in the future. Because there is a need to fit in and look stylish, people will tend to avoid the details and warnings against such types of styles. You need to decide what is important to you: your hair for life, or a temporary hairstyle.

The Psychological Impact of Hair Damage and Loss

Believe me when I say hair loss is devastating, and by the time a person realizes they are losing hair, they have lost 50 percent of their hair already. Hair loss is progressive, so act quickly rather than cover up a problem. Without early treatment, your hair loss will get worse and you will not have a choice but to cover up or shave it all off.

How tight should your hair be braided? If it hurts, it's too tight. The same rule applies with regular braids. Braiding too tight causes a strain on your hair. If you feel your stylist is braiding your hair too tight, SAY SOMETHING! It's your hair. (Do the "eyebrow check" — if you raise your eyebrows and you feel the braids pulling at your scalp, you need to call your stylist back. The oil sheen really won't help this time!

It is believed that there is a link between stress, depression, and hair loss. There are documented cases of people starting to lose hair, anywhere from a few weeks to a few months after a stressful episode in their lives. Of course, hair loss itself is stressful, so it is not always clear which came first, hair loss or stress. According to the American Academy of Dermatology, men and women with androgenetic alopecia have a higher incidence of personality disorders. According to the academy, women with hair loss experience a lack of self-esteem, are introverted, feel less attractive, and are tense in public places.

50 percent of your hair is already lost by the time you realize you're losing hair

- Approximately 30 million women (1 in 4) experience hereditary hair loss or baldness.

- 40 percent of women never expected to face the challenge of hair loss.
- Typically, your hair is at its thickest by age 20; however, your hair gradually begins to thin, shedding more than the normal 40 – 100 strands each day.
- Women who experience hair loss have a disproportionately high rate of fine hair before they lose hair.

Hair loss is an emotional trigger and is an issue of appearance. Severe emotional stress was clear in a recent study of women confronting hair loss:

Most women are highly sensitive to a social expectation that "a woman's hair is her crowning glory." When she perceives that hair loss detracts from the appearance of her "crowning glory," a woman is likely to experience a loss of self-esteem.

Women who have hair loss often perceive that it is not taken seriously by family and friends. Women have less of a support system for hair loss than that which is available to men. Family and friends may commiserate with a man about hair loss and even help him find humor in it. Hair loss (balding) in typical male-pattern alopecia is even an event that is accepted and even expected. Female hair loss is not widely regarded as "normal," even though it occurs frequently. I never met a woman who expected to lose her hair. The psychological effect of hair loss in women is under-appreciated, and perhaps that is due to the lack of public awareness of hair loss in women.

- Female study participants under the age of 50 reported feeling a "severe emotional blow."
- 29 percent admitted feeling scared.
- 47 percent said they were embarrassed.
- 15 percent felt unattractive.
- 28 percent experienced paranoia.

A woman's hair loss should never be overlooked, disregarded, or underestimated. Hair loss should be recognized for the impact it has on a woman's self-esteem and psychological well-being. Additionally, we cannot overlook the fact that hair loss may be an indicator of a much more serious health problem. Since hair is fed directly from the bloodstream, any imbalance within the body can affect the condition and overall well-being of your hair. In other words, know yourself and know your hair.

Don't hesitate to acknowledge changes in your body and in your hair. The cause of the hair loss should be investigated with appropriate medical examination and lab tests until a diagnosis is determined. Hair loss due to the most common causes, such as hereditary female-pattern alopecia, can often be treated effectively; the key is early detection before hair follicles become inactive and are permanently in a resting phase.

5

She Wants Her Body Thinner and Hair Thicker

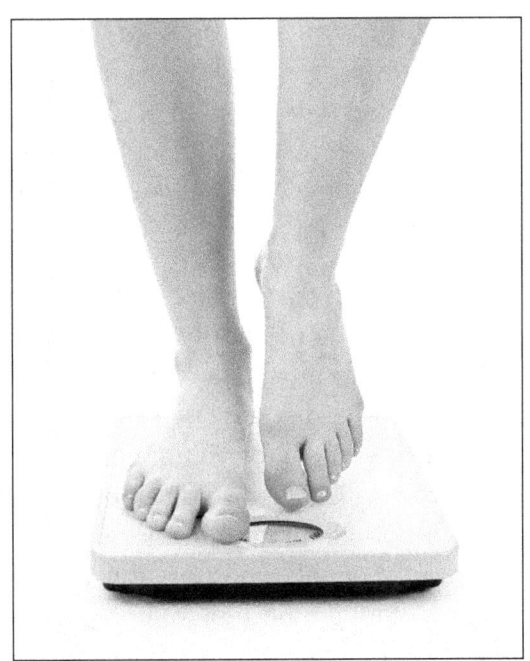

Crash dieting and eating disorders such as **anorexia nervosa** and **bu-limia nervosa** (usually called simply "anorexia" and "bulimia"), and food-related disorders, like binge eating, body image disorders, and food phobias, are becoming more and more common, and now we know that hair loss is linked to these conditions. A lack of essential nutrients in a diet is one of the primary causes of hair loss. Extreme dieting is one form of diet where you compel yourself to starve to lose weight, by drastically curtailing your daily calories. Adequate growth and volume of hair is attained only when you are providing internal nourishment to your body. While you are on a crash diet, the health of your hair is bound to be affected, and hair loss becomes subsequently rapid.

Crash diets are extremely low in calories, which guarantee quick weight loss. However, the side effects of crash dieting could be disastrous. Diets like the lemon water diet, the cabbage soup diet, and the Special K diet are not really useful in the long run. This is because you cannot starve your body permanently. When you resume your normal diet, then you will put on weight randomly. On the other hand, you are depriving yourself of the nutrients that are most required by your body while you are on a crash diet. As already said, the growth of hair is to a large extent dependent upon what you eat, it will tend to thin when you follow a crash diet for a long period.

Hair loss takes place when your body is deficient in proteins and omega-3-fatty acids, which come mostly from animal products and dairy foods. You hardly consume dairy products like milk, butter, or cheese, while following a diet that is extremely low in calories. Omega-3 fatty acids are essential for volume of your hair, while proteins promote hair growth. Chicken and turkey are also sources of niacin that promote blood circulation in the scalp and prevent hair loss. A crash diet mostly entails consumption of small portions of fruits and vegetables. Although these plant compounds contain vitamins, you do not receive them adequately since you are consuming a very small quantity. Similar are the effects of Atkins and cabbage soup diets, where you tend to lose hair after a certain point of time. Eggs are rich sources of biotin that prevent premature graying and hair loss. No matter whether you are reducing consumption of poultry, meat, fruits, or vegetables, it will directly affect your hair, and you will soon observe the damaging effects on your skin as well.

The relationship we all have with our own hair is the ultimate in love/

hate for most of us, and although you may be blaming those bad hair days on harsh winter weather, humidity, or styling products gone wrong, have you considered that it may be your *health* that's really the problem? You can't have healthy hair if you don't have a healthy body, so if you're dealing with hair that's dull, dry, frizzy, flaky, or falling out, it's worth a closer look to make sure it's not due to something bigger than just using the wrong shampoo. From genetics to your current nutritional state, learning to read your hair can tell you a lot about your overall health.

Hair follicles must receive a steady flow of nutrients in order to remain healthy. The follicles receive their nutrients through the blood supply. If circulation is poor, follicles will become malnourished, the root will suffer, and the hair will not grow to its full potential. The increased blood supply helps to nourish and energize the follicles.

If you have a protein deficiency—common with the caloric deprivation of anyone on fad diets or suffering from an eating disorder—it is not unusual to experience severe hair loss. The malnutrition forces the body to conserve protein (the building block of all the body's cells, including the hair) by shutting down hair growth. And since more hair may also be shed—without being replaced—the result can be a noticeable thinning over several months.

Every cell in the body, including the cells needed in normal hair growth, needs protein. Without adequate protein intake, the body cannot efficiently make new hair to replace the hair that has shed. Iron and protein deficiency can be cause for hair loss. See your doctor immediately. Protein deficiency is one of the most common causes of hair loss. Symptoms include splitting and/or falling hair, extreme fatigue, low blood pressure, and brittle nails.

The Iron Factor

An iron deficiency usually is due to blood loss, poor diet, or an inability to absorb enough iron from the foods you eat. Hair problems that are caused by nutritional deficiencies can be corrected by a proper diet. Principal nutrients that are involved include vitamin A, certain B vitamins, the vitamin biotin, vitamin C, copper, iron, zinc, protein, and water.

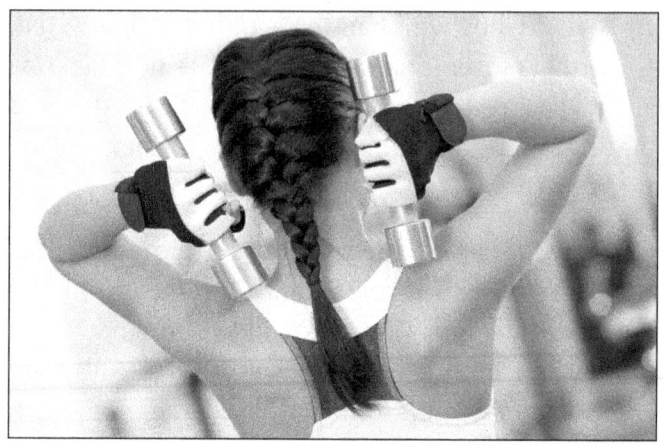

Iron's main job is to carry oxygen in the hemoglobin of red blood cells. Iron deficiency can lead to a condition called anemia, and can also lead to possible hair loss or increased hair shedding.

When you lose blood, you lose iron. If you don't have enough iron stored in your body to make up for the iron loss, you'll develop iron-deficiency anemia.

In women, low iron levels may be due to blood loss from long or heavy menstrual periods or bleeding fibroids in the uterus. Blood loss that occurs during childbirth is another cause for low iron levels in women.

Internal bleeding (bleeding inside the body) also may lead to iron-deficiency anemia. This type of blood loss isn't always obvious, and it may occur slowly. Some causes of internal bleeding are:

- bleeding ulcer, colon polyp, or colon cancer;
- regular use of aspirin or other pain medicines, such as anti-inflammatory drugs (for example, ibuprofen and naproxen); and
- urinary tract bleeding.

Blood loss from severe injuries, surgery, or frequent blood draws also can cause iron-deficiency anemia. This condition will often show it-self in your hairline area. If you've been seemingly trapped in a cycle of your hairline (an area of about 1-2 inches of the circular outer pe-rimeter front to back, similar to a headband) growing then breaking, but never growing to catch up with the rest of your hair length and thickness, this could be the result the above conditions.

Take a Natural Approach

The truth is, eating the right foods will not only help you to feel great, but will you luxurious locks as well. It's true you are what you eat, and this is especially evident with your hair.

Healthy hair depends on the body's ability to construct a proper hair shaft, as well as the health of the skin and follicles. Therefore, good nutrition ensures the best possible environment for building strong, lustrous hair.

However, changing your diet now will affect only *new* growth, not the part of the hair that is already visible. In fact, starting a hair-healthy diet today will mean a more gorgeous head of hair within six months to a year, depending on how fast your hair grows. Hair growth can vary between ¼ inch to 1 inch per month (depending on personal dif-ferences). On average, a person can expect to have about 4 – 6 inches of new growth every year, so it will take about that long to notice the effects of your nutritional changes.

You Really Are What You Eat

Believe it or not your hair is fed and nourished directly from your bloodstream, so a **nutritious diet** provides the fuel to allow hair to thrive. With busy schedules, and poor eating habits, many of us don't get all of the nutrients needed for healthy hair growth through diet alone. The food you eat is digested and absorbed into your body in order to nourish the functioning systems that keep you alive. Your blood flows and is recycled, carrying nutrition to your organs.

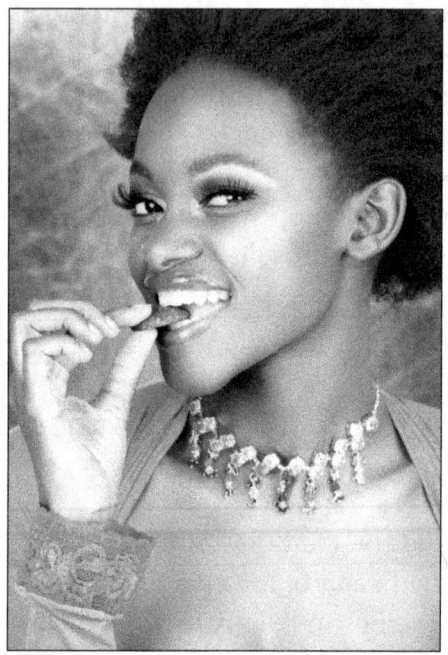

Unfortunately, hair is pretty low on the list of importance to sustain life. Your heart, liver, kidneys, brain, etc., all get a portion of daily nutrition, before hair. For that matter hair, in today's world, has no essential purpose, so if anything is left, it can go to support hair health. Believe me, as you get older, this scenario doesn't get better. This is why natural products for hair growth and hair loss have become so popular and necessary. There are specific vitamins and nutrients that can have a profound effect on your hair's overall health.

Examples of these hair growth products are food supplements, and vitamins like A, zinc, and folic acid. These are important in keeping your hair healthy because they help build and repair cells in the body, especially hair cells. These food supplements have no scientific proof that they cure hair loss problems, but you should know their importance because these are provided in your diet.

Here are some important nutrients for healthy hair and a healthy body:

- **Protein** is an important nutrient because it is the building block of all cells in the body, especially hair cells. Inadequate protein in the diet may result in dry and brittle hair strands.

- You can eat fish, meat, cheese, eggs, and milk to have adequate amounts of protein in your body. Most people get more than enough protein in their diet alone and should not use supplements with protein or amino acids. Only strict vegetarians should supplement protein in their diet.

- *Vitamins* are needed by the body in order to grow healthy hair. These are vitamin A, C, E and all B vitamins like B6 and B12, biotin, folic acid, etc. In addition to these, MSM can be used to naturally lengthen the hair growth phase.

- **Vitamin A** is vital because it prevents the drying and clogging of sebaceous glands, which produces sebum. Sebum is important in lubricating the hair follicles. A deficiency in vitamin A makes your scalp become dry and thick, causing dandruff that could eventually lead to hair loss.

- Vitamin A can be supplied in the diet by eating foods like carrots, sweet potatoes, and liver.

- **B-vitamins—folate, vitamin B-6, vitamin B-12** and **folic acid** — are involved in the creation of red blood cells, which carry oxygen and nutrients to all body cells, including those of the scalp, follicles, and growing hair. Without enough B vitamins, the cells will not thrive, causing shedding, slow growth, or weak hair that is prone to breaking.

- Good sources of vitamin B6 include fortified whole-grain breakfast cereals, garbanzo beans, wild salmon, lean beef, pork tenderloin, chicken breast, white potatoes (w/skin), bananas, and lentils.

- Good sources of Vitamin B12 include shellfish (clams, oysters, crab), wild salmon, fortified whole-grain breakfast cereal, soy milk, trout, lean beef, and low-fat cottage cheese.

▪ Good sources of folate include fortified whole-grain breakfast cereals, lentils, black-eyed peas, soybeans, oatmeal, turnip greens, spinach, green peas, artichokes, okra, beets, parsnips, and broccoli.

▪ **Vitamin C** is important in maintaining collagen in the body. Collagen is essential in keeping your body tissues connected and tightly packed. A deficiency in vitamin C results to hair breakages and split ends.

▪ Good sources of vitamin C are citrus fruits, peppers, broccoli, strawberries, guava, peppers, oranges, grapefruit, pineapple, papayas, lemons, kale, and Brussels sprouts.

▪ **Vitamin E** is responsible for keeping a healthy blood circulation and good supply of oxygen to different parts of the body. A deficiency in this vitamin results in ineffective absorption of fats from the diet.

▪ Vitamin E can be supplied in the body by consuming green leafy vegetables, nuts, grains, and vegetable oils.

▪ **Biotin**, another key ingredient, promotes cell growth, the production of fatty acids, and metabolism of fats and amino acids.

▪ **Minerals** are important micronutrients that must be supplied in the body. Important minerals are **iron, silica,** and **zinc.** Excellent sources of iron are clams, oysters, and liver. Good sources are beef, shrimp, and sardines.

▪ **Silica** is a trace mineral needed by the body. A deficiency in silica can cause hair problems. Foods rich in silica are oats, rice, green leafy vegetables, and strawberries.

- **Zinc** is vital in tissue growth and repair, including hair growth. It also stimulates secretion of oil in the scalp and hair follicles. It also helps keep the oil glands around the hair follicles working properly. Low levels of zinc can cause hair loss, slow growth, and dandruff. Good sources of zinc include oysters, lean beef, crab, ostrich, pork tenderloin, peanut butter, wheat germ, turkey, veal, pumpkin seeds, chicken, and chickpeas.

6

The Link Between Your Health and Your Hair

The Hair Thing Connects with Every Thing!

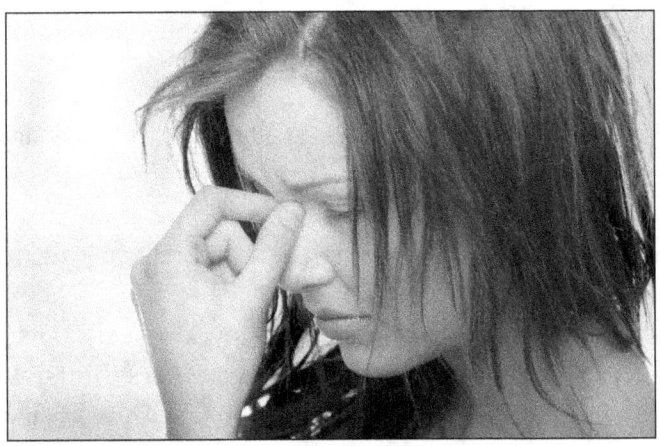

In reality, hair connects with many aspects of your life. The condition of hair, whether it's thinning, breaking, dry, or brittle may be an indicator of other health conditions. The list of conditions includes autoimmune conditions such as Lupus and Crohn's disease, thyroid disorders, hormone imbalance, fibroid anemia, iron deficiency, and many other conditions that would certainly require the attention of a physician, such as diabetes. Just remember your hair is fed directly by your blood supply, so any imbalance within the body will show in the condition of your hair.

Iron deficiency and anemia in women have been shown in several clinical studies to be a frequent cause of hair loss in non-menopausal women 35 to 50. In women the major cause of hair loss before the age of 50 is nutritional, with 30 percent affected. Increased and persistent hair shedding (chronic telogen effluvium) and reduced hair volume are the principal changes occurring. The main cause appears to be depleted iron stores, compromised by an insufficient intake of the essential amino acid l-lysine.

Another study of 153 women with telogen effluvium, conducted from 1995 to 1998, showed that iron deficiency and depletion was the culprit in 72 percent of women. (2)

The most common reasons for iron deficiency due to blood loss include:

- Bleeding in the digestive tract, often due to ulcers and inflammation of the stomach (gastritis).
- Pregnancy: blood loss during and after birth may cause a woman to become iron-deficient, which may result in anemia or hair loss.
- Menstruation: excessively heavy periods can cause an iron deficiency in women, especially when combined with other factors, such as inadequate iron intake. This is often evident when a woman is suffering from enlarged fibroid tumors.
- Severe injuries

A decreased absorption of iron can be caused by medications that reduce stomach acids, lack of stomach acids, chronic diarrhea, and partial removal of the intestines or stomach. Some foods, such as black or pekoe teas, coffee, bran, soybeans, split peas, and dried beans can actually decrease the absorption of iron into the bloodstream.

Another cause of low iron might include decreased iron intake or lack of iron in the diet. Good sources of iron include lean red meat, steamed clams, Cream of Wheat, dried fruit, soybeans, tofu, broccoli, and spinach.

Ferritin is a protein that stores iron in the body. The serum ferritin level — the amount of ferritin in your blood — is directly proportional to the amount of iron stored in your body. Ferritin is a more accurate monitor of long-term body iron status than the blood iron level, which varies with diet.

Serum ferritin concentrations provide a good assessment of an individual's iron status. What level of serum ferritin to provide for those with increased hair shedding has yet to be definitively established. The role of the essential amino acid l-lysine in hair loss also appears to be important. *To determine if you have iron deficiency, doctors will most likely conduct a ferritin test.* The amount of ferritin in the blood indicates how much iron the body has in reserve.

Solution and Treatment

Hair loss in women and men due to iron deficiency can be easily resolved in most cases with modification of the daily diet to include more foods rich in vitamins, which can include red meat, dried fruit, broccoli, raisins, clams, oysters, and spinach. Iron supplement pills and the amino acid l-lysine can also eliminate the problem.

The RDA (Recommended Daily Allowance) for Iron is 15 mg for women and 18 mg for men.

Anemia and Iron

The body needs iron to make hemoglobin. If not enough iron is available, hemoglobin production is limited, which in turns affects the production of red blood cells. A decrease in the normal amount of hemoglobin and red blood cells circulating in the bloodstream is known as anemia. Because red blood cells are needed to carry oxygen throughout the body, anemia results in less oxygen reaching the cells and tissues, affecting their function. It is important to note that not all cases of iron deficiency result in anemia.

What You May Not Know About Diabetes and Hair Loss

Many people who suffer from diabetes don't know they have it. Sudden hair loss can be one of the first noticeable symptoms of diabetes.

There are two types of diabetes, and both involve insulin, which is produced by the pancreas to break down carbohydrates during digestion. This disease can have many adverse effects on your body, including hair loss.

Diabetes and Hair Loss Can Be Related

Why is diabetes one of the causes of hair loss? Your body has certain metabolic cycles, and one of these is the hair growth cycle. An individual hair will grow for several years and then enter a resting phase before being shed. In a healthy person, this hair re-grows. Diabetes affects the normal metabolic cycles of your body, including the hair growth cycle. If this cycle is disrupted, hair that is shed normally may not re-grow right away, or it may not re-grow at all.

Other Ways Diabetes Can Affect Hair Growth

Diabetes can also affect hair growth in these ways:

- This disease weakens your immune system. The result is increased susceptibility to infections, including scalp infections, which can cause hair loss.
- Diabetes adversely affects the circulatory system, causing problems all over your body, including your scalp. Hair follicles that don't get enough nutrients because of circulatory problems can't produce new hairs, and the follicles may even die from lack of nutrition.
- Diabetes is a hormonal disease, disrupting other hormone levels in your body. Hair loss in women is often caused by hormonal imbalances.
- Skin rashes and thyroid conditions are often seen with diabetes, and these conditions also affect the hair growth cycle.

If you have already been diagnosed with diabetes, and you're taking medication to control it, be aware the some of these medications can cause hair loss, too. Your doctor may need to change or adjust your prescription.

If you have only one of these symptoms, it probably isn't anything to worry about. But if you're struggling with two or more, even if hair loss is not a problem, you could have diabetes and not know it. See your doctor right away for a thorough check-up.

Autoimmune Diseases can Wreak Havoc on your Hair

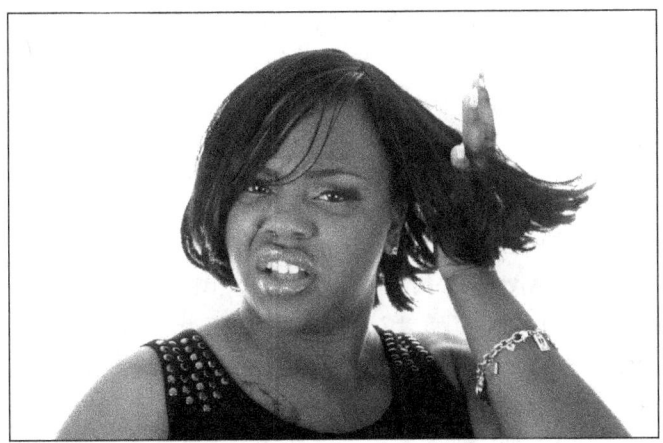

Autoimmune conditions wreak havoc on the body. Did you know that your hair will show signs of the underlying problem very early on?

According to AARDA (American Autoimmune Related Diseases Association), "the term "autoimmune disease" refers to a varied group of more than 80 serious, chronic illnesses that involve almost every human organ system. In all of these diseases the underlying problem is similar and the body's immune system becomes misdirected, attacking the very organs it was designed to protect.

These diseases happen when our body fails to recognize its own part and attacks itself with antibodies in response. It's like our body finding a normal everyday cell and thinking, "Oh! I found a diseased cell. Let's attack and kill it." Now imagine how many normal cells your body has and what will happen when each of them is treated as a diseased cell.

The autoimmune response sets off a series of symptoms throughout the body and directly impacts the condition of the hair, including thinning, color loss, dryness, changes in texture, and hair loss. These symptoms are common features of autoimmune disease. Of these, hair loss can be the most devastating. Overall, hair loss can have many medical causes including hormonal imbalances, medication effects, and autoimmune diseases. Among the autoimmune diseases that cause hair loss or baldness, alopecia areata is the most common. Alopecia areata may affect small localized scalp patches, or it may affect the entire body. Treatment is available for alopecia areata although, in general, the more hair lost, the less successful the treatment will be.

Autoimmune Disease and Hair loss

Alopecia Areata (AA): When most people think of autoimmune hair loss, AA is typically the first thing that comes to mind. This condition is known as the reason that Princess Caroline of Monaco temporarily lost her hair. The condition most often presents itself in hair loss that is defined by bald spots that are round and patchy. Often, the hair around the patches is totally normal, but the round patchy areas are smooth and sometimes completely bald.

There is a lot of controversy over what actually causes **alopecia areata**. Most agree that it is autoimmune in nature, but some believe that it is aggravated by stress, allergies, or viruses. Treatment is often oral steroids, corticosteroid injections, or experimental stimulation of the scalp with herbs like rosemary and lavender.

Areata Universalis is another condition that goes hand in hand with AA. In this case, you will often have hair loss over the entire body including the whole head (often total baldness) as well as other areas like eyelashes, eyebrows, pubic hair, the beard area, the underarms, etc. Sometimes when this process is ongoing, you'll see "exclamation point hairs." These are hairs that are broken off and are tapered so that they are much narrower the closer you get the scalp. They flare out on the broken ends.

Scarring alopecia is a potentially permanent and irreversible destruction of hair follicles and their replacement with scar tissue.

Most forms of scarring alopecia first occur as small patches of hair loss that may expand with time. In some cases the hair loss is gradual, without noticeable symptoms, and may go unnoticed for a long time. In other instances, the hair loss is associated with severe itching, burning, and pain and is rapidly progressive.

The scarring alopecia patches usually look a little different from alopecia areata in that the edges of the bald patches look more "ragged." The destruction of the hair follicle occurs below the skin surface, so there may not be much to actually see on the scalp's skin surface other than patchy hair loss. Affected areas may be smooth and clean, or may have redness, scaling, increased or decreased pigmentation, or may have raised blisters with fluids or pus coming from the affected area.

It is difficult to diagnose a scarring alopecia just from the pattern of the hair loss and the nature of the scalp skin. Often when scarring alopecia is suspected, one or more skin biopsies are done to confirm the diagnosis and help identify the particular form of scarring alopecia. A small biopsy is taken and examined under a microscope. A pathologist or dermatologist will look for destruction of the hair follicles, scar tissue deep in the skin, and the presence and location of inflammation in relation to the hair follicles.

Often, the early stages of a scarring alopecia will have inflammatory cells around the hair follicles, which, many researchers believe, induces the destruction of the hair follicles and development of scar tissue. However, there is some argument about this among dermatologists as sometimes a biopsy from a scarring-alopecia-affected individual shows very little inflammation.

Scarring alopecia almost always burns out. The bald patches stop expanding and any inflammation, itching, burning, or pain goes away. In this end stage another skin biopsy usually shows no inflammation around hair follicles. Bald areas usually have no more hair follicles. Sometimes, though, hair follicles — at least those at the periphery of a bald patch — are not completely destroyed and can re-grow, but often all that is left are just a few longitudinal scars deep in the skin to show where the hair follicles once were.

Treatment Options

Scarring alopecia can involve a lot of damage and permanent hair loss. For this reason treatment of scarring alopecia should be quite aggressive. The nature of treatment varies depending on the particular diagnosis. Scarring alopecias that involve mostly lymphocyte inflammation of hair follicles, such as lichen planopilaris and pseudopelade, are generally treated with corticosteroids in topical creams and by injection into the affected skin.

Once a scarring alopecia has reached the burnt-out stage and there has been no more hair loss for a few years, bald areas can be either surgically removed if they are not too big or the bald patches can be transplanted with hair follicles taken from unaffected areas.

Autoimmune conditions in which localized or diffused hair loss can occur include: systemic lupus, Hashimoto's thyroiditis, Graves' disease, and postmenopausal frontal alopecia. In systemic lupus, malar rash can cause scarring of the scalp that leads to permanent hair loss. Hashimoto's thyroiditis causes hair to coarsen and become dry, contributing to hair loss, which is seen in more than 50 percent of patients. In Graves' disease, hair tends to become fine and brittle with a reluctance to hold curl and a tendency toward hair loss. Hair loss is reported in 20-40 percent of patients with Graves' disease.

Here is a partial checklist of frequently noticed symptoms of the most common autoimmune conditions:

- Alopecia Areata
  - » Hair loss, round bald patches on the scalp
- Alopecia Totalis, Hashimoto's Hypothyroidism, Graves' Disease / Hyperthyroidism, Lupus
  - » Hair loss, loss of facial and scalp hair
- Hashimoto's Hypothyroidism, Graves' Disease/ Hyperthyroidism, Polycystic Ovary Syndrome (PCOS)
  - » Male-pattern baldness
- Cushing's Disease, Polycystic Ovary Syndrome (PCOS)
  - » Excess hair growth on the face, neck, chest, abdomen, and thighs, in women
- Hashimoto's Hypothyroidism
  - » Loss of hair in outer eyebrow
- Hashimoto's Hypothyroidism, Graves' Disease/ Hyperthyroidism
  - » Hair is rough, coarse dry, breaking, brittle

TREATMENT

In endocrine disorders, correcting the hormone imbalance helps restore hair growth and improve its texture. Hair growth also responds to dietary changes. In particular, adding high-quality protein to the diet can help restore hair growth. When hair loss suddenly increases it can reflect inadequate dietary protein or malabsorption, a condition of poor nutrient absorption from dietary sources. Malabsorption is common in thyroid disorders, Crohn's disease, pernicious anemia, and celiac disease.

A nutrient-rich diet with adequate protein and dietary supplements, particularly vitamin B complex, can help promote hair growth. Biotin promotes hair and scalp health and can help prevent hair loss. Excellent sources of biotin include nuts, brown rice, brewer's yeast, and oats. Iron deficiency (confirmed by blood tests) can also cause hair loss, and restoring iron levels can reverse hair loss. Foods rich in iron include green leafy vegetables, leeks, cashews, berries, dried fruits, and figs. Vitamin C is necessary for iron absorption. Eating citrus foods after an iron-rich meal helps absorption. Vitamin E, zinc, and essential fatty acids, such as flaxseed and fish oils, are also important for hair growth. A greens formula containing chlorella, spirulina, barley, and wheatgrass also promotes hair growth.

Rosemary essential oil used as a scalp massage ingredient or added to shampoo can help hair growth by improving the scalp circulation.

Stay tuned in to noticeable changes in your body and your hair. Be careful not to ignore nature's signs of health imbalance. Subtle or drastic changes should be mentioned to your professional health care provider. Remember, early detection is always the key to a better outcome.

Lupus and Hair Loss: Probably the second most common autoimmune disorder known to cause hair issues is lupus. Often someone with this condition is affected with a rash that can affect the scalp and cause scarring, which can lead to temporary or permanent hair loss.

Thyroid Issues: Graves' Disease and Hashimoto's Thyroiditis: Many people who think of thyroid issues and hair loss are aware of hypothyroidism, but many are not aware of the autoimmune thyroid issues. The first of these is Graves' disease where you will generally see the hair become much finer and you'll see more pronounced loss. The texture just becomes a lot more limp and unable to hold a style. The strands can become lighter in color also. The opposite is true with Hashimoto's. In this instance, the hair becomes very coarse and dry, but hair loss is accelerated nonetheless.

Lesser-Known Autoimmune Disorders That May Affect the Hair: In truth, almost any disorder that has an autoimmune component can affect the hair or cause thinning, shedding, or loss. This includes things like rheumatoid arthritis, intestinal cystitis, and fibromyalgia, (although not everyone agrees that these two fall into this category), celiac disease, and Guillain-Barre syndrome, to name only a few.

Inflammation-Lessening Drugs and Hair Loss: Many of the drugs that are given for these disorders are given to reduce the inflammatory process and this actually seems to fit quite nicely with hair loss treatment, as there is almost always an inflammation component to it. However, many of the steroids often used have the unfortunate side effect of more shedding or loss, so often the patient is left wondering if it's the disorder that is affecting their hair or the medication that is being used to treat it. It's often prudent to focus on a healthy diet and healthy natural ways to support a healthy scalp and reduce inflammation while stimulating healthy re-growth.

Thyroid Disease Causes: Many people notice rapid hair loss as a symptom of their hyperthyroidism or hypothyroidism. It's estimated that 59 million Americans have a thyroid problem, but the majority don't even know it yet. The thyroid, a butterfly-shaped gland located in the neck, is the master gland of metabolism. When your thyroid doesn't function, it can affect every aspect of your health, and in particular, weight, depression, and energy levels.

Since undiagnosed thyroid problems can dramatically increase your risk of obesity, heart disease, depression, anxiety, hair loss, sexual dysfunction, infertility, and a host of other symptoms and health problems, it's important that you don't go undiagnosed. Some people actually say this is the worst symptom of their thyroid problem — thinning hair, large amounts falling out in the shower or sink, often accompanied by changes in the hair's texture, making it dry, coarse, or easily tangled. Interestingly, some people have actually written to tell me that their thyroid problem was initially discovered by their hairdresser, who noticed the change.

7

Can Prescription Drugs Cause Hair Loss?

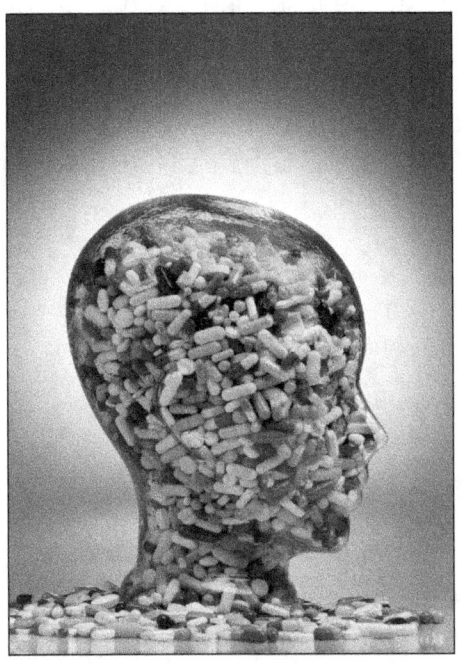

Prescription Drugs can often cause temporary hair loss or trigger the onset of male- and female-pattern baldness, and even cause permanent hair loss. Note that the drugs listed here do not include those used in chemotherapy and radiation for cancer treatment.

Your doctor may not mention hair loss as a side effect of some drugs, so don't forget to do your own research and read the drug manufacturer's complete warnings. Your pharmacist can provide you with this information even before you fill a prescription.

Many pill and medication guidebooks (sold in bookstores and pharmacies) are also excellent sources of complete information about prescription drugs. If your doctor prescribes any of the following drugs, ask if one that does not have hair loss as a possible side effect can be substituted.

The drugs are listed by category, according to the conditions they treat, then by brand name first, followed by the drug's generic name in parentheses. In some categories, individual drugs are not listed. For these conditions, you will want to discuss the possibility of hair loss as a side effect of using any of the drugs that treat that particular condition, since many do contribute to hair loss.

Acne
All drugs derived from vitamin A as treatments for acne or other conditions, including Accutane (isotretinoin)

Blood
Anticoagulants (blood thinners), including:

- Panwarfin (warfarin sodium)
- Sofarin (warfarin sodium)
- Coumadin (warfarin sodium)
- Heparin injections

Cholesterol
Cholesterol-lowering drugs, including:

- Atronid-S (clofibrate)
- Lopid (gemfibrozil)

Convulsions/ Epilepsy
- ▪ Anticonvulsants, including:
- ▪ Tridone (trimethadione)

Depression
- ▪ Antidepression drugs, including:
- ▪ Prozac (fluoxetine hydrochloride)
- ▪ Zoloft (sertraline hydrochloride)
- ▪ Paxil (paroxetine)
- ▪ Anafranil (clomipramine)
- ▪ Janimine (imipramine)
- ▪ Tofranil (imipramine)
- ▪ Tofranil PM (imipramine)
- ▪ Adapin (doxepin)
- ▪ Sinequan (doxepin)
- ▪ Surmontil (trimipramine)
- ▪ Pamelor (nortriptyline)
- ▪ Ventyl (nortriptyline)
- ▪ Elavin (amitriptyline)
- ▪ Endep (amitriptyline)
- ▪ Norpramin (desipramine)
- ▪ Pertofrane (desipramine)
- ▪ Vivactil (protriptyline hydrochloride)
- ▪ Asendin (amoxapine)
- ▪ Haldol (haloperidol)

Diet
- ▪ Amphetamines

Fungus
- ▪ Antifungals

Glaucoma

The beta-blocker drugs, including:

- Timoptic Eye Drops (timolol)
- Timoptic Ocudose (timolol)
- Timoptic XC (timolol)

Gout

- Lopurin (allopurinol)
- Zyloprim (allopurinol)

Heart

Many drugs prescribed for the heart, including those known as the beta blockers, which are also used to treat high blood pressure, and include:

- Tenormin (atenolol)
- Lopressor (metoprolol)
- Corgard (nadolol)
- Inderal and Inderal LA (propanolol)
- Blocadren (timolol)

High Blood Pressure

See Above list of beta blockers under "Heart"

Hormonal Conditions

All hormone-containing drugs and drugs prescribed for hormone-related, reproductive, male-specific, and female-specific conditions and situations have the potential to cause hair loss, including:

- Birth control pills
- Hormone-replacement therapy (HRT) for women (estrogen or progesterone)
- Male androgenic hormones and all forms of testosterone

- Anabolic steriods
- Prednisone and other steroids

Inflammation

Many anti-inflammatory drugs, including those prescribed for localized pain, swelling and injury.

- Arthritis drugs
- Nonsteroidal Anti-Inflammatory Drugs including:
- Naprosyn (naproxen)
- Anaprox (naproxen)
- Anaprox DS (naproxen)
- Indocin (indomethacin)
- Indocin SR (indomethacin)
- Clinoril (sulindac)
- An anti-inflammatory that is also used as a chemotherapy drug:
- Methotrexate (MTX)
- Rheumatex (methotrexate)
- Folex (methotrexate)

Parkinson's Disease

- Levadopa / L-dopa (dopar, larodopa)

Thyroid Disorders

- Many of the drugs used to treat the thyroid

Ulcer

Many of the drugs used to treat indigestion, stomach difficulties, and ulcers, including over-the-counter dosages and prescription dosages.

- Tagamet (cimetidine)
- Zantac (ranitidine)
- Pepcid (famotidine)

Chemotherapy and Hair Loss:

You might not think about how important your hair is until you face losing it. And, if you have cancer and are about to undergo chemotherapy, the chance of hair loss is very real. Both men and women report hair loss as one of the side effects they fear most after being diagnosed with cancer.

Whether or not you have hair loss from your chemotherapy depends mostly on the type and dose of medication you receive. But whether you can maintain a healthy body image after hair loss depends a lot on your attitude and the support of your friends and family.

Chemotherapy and hair loss: Why does it occur?

Chemotherapy drugs are powerful medications that attack rapidly growing cancer cells. Unfortunately, these drugs also attack other rapidly growing cells in your body — including those in your hair roots.

Chemotherapy may cause hair loss all over your body — not just on your scalp. Sometimes your eyelashes, eyebrows, armpit, pubic and other body hair also falls out. Some chemotherapy drugs are more likely than others to cause hair loss, and different doses can cause anything from a mere thinning to complete baldness. Talk to your doctor or nurse about the medication you'll be taking. Your doctor or nurse can tell you what to expect.

Fortunately, most of the time hair loss from chemotherapy is temporary. You can expect to re-grow a full head of hair six months to a year after your treatment ends, though your hair may temporarily be a different shade or texture.

Chemotherapy and hair loss: What should you expect?

Hair usually begins falling out 10 to 14 days after you start treatment. It could fall out very quickly in clumps or gradually. You'll likely notice accumulations of loose hair on your pillow, in your hairbrush, or in your sink or shower drain.

Your hair loss will continue throughout your treatment and up to a month afterward. Whether your hair thins or you become completely bald will depend on your treatment. Generally, you can lose about 50 percent of your hair before it's noticeable to other people.

It takes about four to six weeks for your hair to recover from chemotherapy. In general, you can expect about a quarter inch of growth each month.

When your hair starts to grow back, it will probably be slightly different from the hair you lost. But, the difference is usually temporary. Your new hair might have a different texture or color. It might be curlier than it was before, or it could be gray until the cells that control the pigment in your hair begin functioning again.

Chemotherapy and hair loss: Can hair loss be prevented?

No treatment exists that can guarantee your hair won't fall out during or after chemotherapy. The best way to deal with impending hair loss is to plan ahead and focus on making yourself comfortable with your appearance before, during, and after your cancer treatment.

Several treatments have been investigated as possible ways to prevent hair loss, but none has been absolutely effective, including:

- **Scalp hypothermia (cryotherapy).** During chemotherapy, ice packs or similar devices are placed on the head to slow blood flow to your scalp. This way, chemotherapy drugs are less likely to have an effect on the scalp. Studies of scalp hypothermia have found it works somewhat in the majority of people who have tried it. However, the procedure also causes a small risk of cancer recurring in the scalp, as this area doesn't receive the same dose of chemotherapy as the rest of the body. Most people who try this procedure find it to be uncomfortable and very cold.

- **Minoxidil (Rogaine).** Applying minoxidil — a drug approved for pattern hair loss in men and women — to the scalp before and during chemotherapy isn't likely to prevent hair loss, although some research shows it may speed up hair re-growth. More research is needed to understand whether minoxidil is effective in re-growing hair after cancer treatment

Hair loss generally can't be prevented or controlled, but it can be managed. Take the following steps throughout your treatment to minimize the frustration and anxiety associated with hair loss.

Before Chemotherapy Treatment

- **Be gentle to your hair.** Get in the habit of being kind to your hair. Don't bleach, color, or perm your hair — this can weaken it. Air-dry your hair as much as possible and avoid heating devices such as curling irons and hot rollers. Strengthening your hair now might make it more likely to stay in your head a little longer during treatment.

- **Consider cutting your hair.** Short hair tends to look fuller than long hair. So as your hair falls out, it won't be as noticeable if you have short hair. Also, if you have long hair, going short might help you make a better transition to total hair loss.

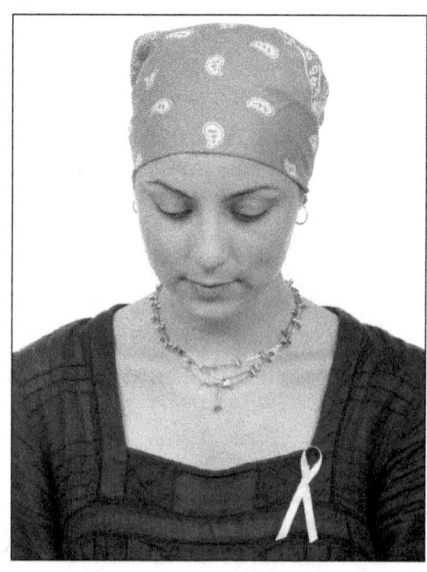

- **Plan ahead for a head covering.** Now is the time to start thinking about wigs, scarves, or other head coverings. Whether you choose to wear a head covering to conceal your hair loss is up to you. But it's easier to plan for it now rather than later. Ask your doctor to write a prescription for a wig, the cost of which may be covered by your health insurance.

During Chemotherapy Treatment

- **Baby your remaining hair.** Continue your gentle hair strategies throughout your chemotherapy treatment. Try using a satin pillowcase, which is less likely to attract and catch fragile hair. Use a soft brush. Wash your hair only as often as necessary. Consider using a gentle shampoo. Stay away from shampoos with strong detergents and chemicals that can dry out your scalp, including salicylic acid, alcohol, and strong fragrances.

- **Consider shaving your head.** Some report that scalps feel itchy, sensitive, and irritated during their treatment and while their hair is falling out. Shaving your head can reduce the irritation and save the embarrassment of shedding. Some men shave their heads because they feel it looks better than the patchy hair loss they might be experiencing. Also, a shaved head might be easier for securing a wig or hairpiece.

- **Protect your scalp.** If your head is going to be exposed to the sun or to cold air, protect it with sunscreen or a head covering. Your scalp may be sensitive as you go through treatment, so extreme cold or sunshine can easily irritate it even more. Having no hair or having less hair can make you feel cold, so a head covering may make you more comfortable.

After Chemotherapy Treatment

- **Continue gentle hair care.** Your new hair growth will be especially fragile and vulnerable to the damage caused by styling products and heating devices. Hold off on coloring or bleaching your new hair for at least six months. Besides damaging new hair, processing could irritate your sensitive scalp.

▪ **Be patient.** It's likely that your hair will come back slowly and that it might not look normal right away. Growth takes time, and it also takes time to repair the damage caused by your cancer treatment.

Covering your head as your hair falls out is a purely personal decision. For many women, hair is associated with femininity and health, so they choose to maintain that look by wearing a wig. Others choose hats and scarves. Still others choose not to cover their heads at all.

Ask your doctor or a hospital social worker about resources in your area to help you find the best head covering for you. Look Good... Feel Better is a free program that provides hair and beauty makeovers and tips to women with cancer. These classes are offered throughout the United States and in several other countries. Many classes are offered through local chapters of the American Cancer Society. Look Good...Feel Better also offers classes for teens with cancer, as well as a website especially for men.

Radiation therapy also can cause hair loss

Radiation therapy also attacks quickly growing cells in your body, but unlike chemotherapy, it affects only the specific area where treatment is concentrated. If you have radiation to your head, you'll likely lose the hair on your head.

Your hair usually begins growing back after your treatments end. But whether it grows back to its original thickness and fullness depends on your treatment. Different types of radiation and different doses will have different effects on your hair. Higher doses of radiation can cause permanent hair loss. Talk to your doctor about what dose you'll be receiving so that you'll know what to expect.

Radiation therapy also affects your skin. The treatment area is likely to be red and may look sunburned or tanned. If your radiation treatment is to your head, it's a good idea to cover your head with a protective hat or scarf because your skin will be sensitive to cold and sunlight. Wigs and other hairpieces might irritate your scalp.

8

Birth Control — Testosterone and Other Hormonal Hair Bandits

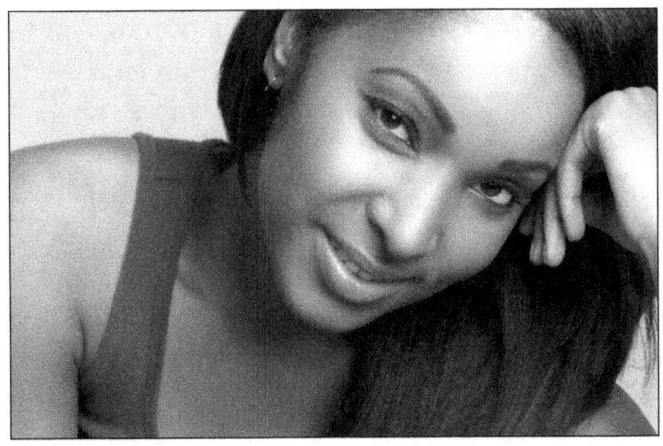

In women, hair loss can be triggered by a multitude of conditions and circumstances. One cause not to be overlooked is hormonal imbalance. In women this is crucial because estrogen is a major driver of hair growth, but there is a delicate balance that must be maintained. Too much or not enough estrogen can create major hair loss issues in women of all ages. Women using birth control, and especially those who have a history of hair loss in their family, should be aware of the potentially devastating effects of birth control pills, patches, and shots on normal hair growth.

The American Hair Loss Association recommends that all women interested in using oral contraceptives for the prevention of conception should use only low-androgen index birth control pills, and if there is a strong predisposition for genetic hair loss in your family, it may be best to consider non-hormonal forms of birth control.

Of course, birth control pills contain progesterone and estrogen, so you'd think they'd be great for your hair. Unfortunately, they can cause thinning in some women. "The progesterone component can break down into a male-like hormone in the body," according to Dr. Neil Sadic, M.D., a New York-based dermatologist. So if your hair seems limper since you started the Pill, ask your doctor about switching to a low-progesterone dose.

Hair loss after pregnancy is a very common occurrence. As distressing as it can be, especially with the concerns of having a new baby, the hair loss is simply indicating that your hair is slowly but surely returning to its normal condition.

There are two hair growth phases that we need to take into account when looking at hair loss after pregnancy.

There is a growth period that can last anywhere from 4 years to 7 years. This is called the "anagen" phase, with hair growing approximately 1-2 cm a month.

After each growth period there is a resting phase known as The "telogen" phase. This period of the hair growth cycle lasts for 3-4 months typically, whereupon the growth phase signals the beginning of a new cycle.

What happens during this part of the cycle is that older hair falls out due to the new hair growing and pushing it out of the follicle. In normal conditions it is normal to lose up to 100 hairs per day.

Of course not all follicles go into the rest or growth period simultaneously. To keep the hair growth and loss balanced and under control, some follicles are in a growth period while others are resting.

The hormonal situation in a woman's body while she is pregnant

keeps the hair in a strong growth phase. You may notice how a pregnant women's hair looks so healthy and thick. This is due to the fact
that she is not losing hair that she would normally be losing, and so
the density of her hair increases during her pregnancy. So, not only
do you have above-average normal hair growth during pregnancy,
you also do not lose hair during pregnancy that you normally would.

However, once the child is born, dramatic changes in the hormonal
system occur. Part of this rapid change is that all hair follicles simultaneously go into a resting period. The resulting after-pregnancy hair
loss can be extreme.

High levels of the female hormone progesterone and estrogen kick in
while a woman is carrying the baby and create an unusually thick and
healthy head of hair. Those hormones drop off after the baby is born
and hormone levels begin to return to normal. A woman may lose a
frightening amount of hair 1 to 3 months later. 90 to 100 percent of
lost hair should grow back over the next several months, depending
on general health and nutrition. If the fallout of hair does not turn
around within a reasonable amount of time, consult with you doctor.

Some will argue that stress does not cause female hair loss. The stress
and emotional upheaval that occurs with the arrival of a new baby
can certainly exacerbate an already disturbed hormonal system,
leading to an even greater amount of hair loss after pregnancy. As if
that wasn't enough for our new mom, from a nutritional perspective
breast-feeding can severely deplete a woman's nutritional reserves,
leading to the likelihood of even greater hair loss after pregnancy.
There is nothing that can be done to speed up the resting post-preg-
nancy hair growth period. After-pregnancy hair loss is just part of a
normal pregnancy cycle.

Taking care of you hair with appropriate hair care products will help.
Perhaps this is the time to try out a new hairstyle.

Be aware of what you eat, making sure you get enough nutrients
to give yourself all you need, as well as the baby, while you are
breast-feeding.

And, above all else, don't worry. Remember that hair loss after pregnancy is a normal part of the proceedings. Take care of yourself and your baby, and your hair will be back as good as ever in a few months' time.

Menopause: What Momma Never Told You

While it may be more common among men, hair loss in women isn't as rare as you might think. It's estimated that hair loss affects 1 in 5 women.

Hair loss in aging women is largely attributed to hormonal imbalance, as it is in men, and is one of the lesser-known and less-common symptoms of menopause. Hair loss is not as prevalent in women because women have more estrogen than men, and that in turn helps balance out the effects of androgens, namely dihydrotestosterone (DHT), that typically lead to female hair loss. The rate of hair growth slows. Expect change every 10 years after 25 years old. For women, hair growth is at its peak in your early twenties, which coincides with your estrogen levels also being at their peak. Remember, hair growth is tied to and driven by estrogen levels.

The hair strands become smaller and have less pigment, so the thick coarse hair of a young adult eventually becomes thin, fine, and light-colored hair. Many hair follicles stop producing new hairs altogether.

About a quarter of men begin to show signs of baldness by the time they are 30 years old, and about two-thirds of men have significant baldness by age 60. Men develop a typical pattern of baldness associated with the male hormone testosterone (male-pattern baldness). Hair may be lost at the temples or at the top of the head.

Women may also develop a typical pattern of hair loss as they age (female-pattern baldness). The hair becomes less dense all over and the scalp may become visible.

Body and facial hair are also lost, but the hairs that remain may become coarser. Some women may notice a loss of body hair, but may find that they have coarse facial hair, especially on the chin and around the lips. Men may find the hair of their eyebrows, ears, and nose becoming longer and coarser.

Hair is considered the crowning glory of women. The thickness and the length of the hair usually help in making women look more attractive and younger. Looking at the perspective of evolution, early men looked for mates with long and thick hair because it was an indication of a woman's reproductive and general health. Unfortunately, when a woman reaches menopause, her hair starts to thin. Hair loss is actually one of the symptoms of menopause. However, this is not so much addressed and given attention because it is eclipsed by the more irritating and baffling menopausal symptoms such as hot flashes, mood swings, and weight gain. Moreover, hair loss is often more associated with and rampant in males. Actually, hair loss during and after menopause is more common than most people think it is. In fact, about 50 percent of women experience pattern baldness and hair loss during menopause, while roughly 67 percent experience it after menopause.

You probably know menopause is that time when your ovaries stop producing estrogen. Menopause can occur at any time during your adult years, but most commonly happens during your late 40s to mid-50s. Yet regardless of when it happens, menopause signals the end of your reproductive years, meaning no more of this, including not having to worry about birth control and never suffering from menstrual cramps again. Menopause is not, however, so fabulous for your hair. That's because estrogen protects you against hair loss. Without estrogen, your locks may grow noticeably thinner.

For those of you genetically predisposed toward female-pattern hair loss, menopause is when you'll learn whether or not you're going to be affected. This also has to do with the sudden lack of hair-helping estrogen.

Another symptom of aging hair is sebum production (natural oils). Sebum production will slow down considerably and your hair may grow drier. Most humans experience thinning hair with age. By thinning, I don't mean obvious balding. If you are prone to that, now is the time it will start happening. I simply mean that you will have less hair than you did in your youth. That's because as we age, our hair spends less time in the anagen — or growth — stage, and more time in the catagen (transition) and the telogen (resting) stages. At this point, there should be no great hair surprises for you. Instead, with each decade expect a gradual decrease in sebum production and a gradual increase in graying and thinning.

Link Between Menopause and Hair Loss

All women produce a negligible amount of testosterone. However, the effects of this male sex hormone are not evident physically because the high levels of estrogen, a female sex hormone, in a woman's body counteract the effects of testosterone. During and after menopause, however, women experience a sharp decline in the production of estrogen. As a result, testosterone, with the help of a certain enzyme, produces more DHT, which is known to be the cause of hair loss and pattern baldness in women. You may also notice more facial hair growth as the result of less estrogen to counteract the effects of testosterone in the body.

Why Is Estrogen So Important for Hair Growth?

Estrogen is a female sex hormone that is dominant in women, but it can also be found in men in much lesser quantities. Estrogen is a huge driver of hair growth in women and is at the core of many feminine characteristics:

- decelerates height growth
- promotes breast enlargement
- promotes hair growth
- reduces muscle mass

Estrogen contributes greatly to the production of better skin, nails, and hair.

While the male hormone testosterone converts into DHT when there is not sufficient estrogen to balance hormones, this can cause your hair follicles to stop producing hair. If you have normal levels of estrogen in your body, you can rest assured your risk of facing female-pattern baldness is much lower for the early part of your adulthood.

Estrogen and Hair Loss

As you get older in life, or during menopause, your estrogen levels will drop. This can result in what we call a hormonal imbalance. One of the effects of this imbalance is that with the reduction of estrogen, it paves the way for the male hormone testosterone, which converts into DHT to flood the hair follicles.

However, do keep in mind that not all hormonal imbalances are related to estrogen; some can be caused by other diseases such as thyroid problems. Without the adequate presence of estrogen in your body, you might be facing a hair loss condition as your hair is exposed to the effects of DHT. Keep in mind that estrogen and hair loss in women are directly related to each other.

Can You Increase Estrogen Levels?

We have options where estrogen and hair loss are concerned. There are solutions you can choose from to help the situation. Most of these treatments are mainly to stabilize your hormone levels. It's best if you consult your doctor before beginning any treatments.

Some of these treatments are:

- Topical estrogenic products
- Hormone Replacement Therapy
- Estrogen pills
- Food that is high in estrogens (chicken, eggs, etc.)

An increase in estrogen levels is proven to be beneficial for reducing hair loss. Nevertheless, research indicates that in some women, the excess of estrogen can promote various diseases such as breast cancer, as the cancerous cells thrive on estrogen to grow.

As for men, if you increase your estrogen levels, you are actually promoting female characteristics into your body, which I wouldn't recommend, (unless it is for another purpose).

Testosterone (androgen) is a hormone found primarily in males and in reduced amounts in females, though the amount can increase as women approach menopause. Testosterone itself has only limited negative effects on the hair follicles. However, when testosterone reaches the oil glands in the hair follicles, it comes in contact with the enzyme 5-alpha-reductase. 5-alpha-reductase is directly responsible for the conversion of testosterone into dihydrotestosterone (DHT). The enzyme 5-alpha-reductase is produced in the prostate, adrenal glands, and scalp skin. Formation of dihydrotestosterone is a factor for baldness in both men and women, and can be termed as DHT Hair Loss.

DHT (and perhaps other androgens) causes hair follicles to shrink and enter a permanent dormant state. DHT triggers synthesis of transforming growth factor-beta2 (TGF-beta2), which suppresses epithelial cell proliferation and eventually leads to apoptotic cell death. TGF-beta2 is directly responsible for significant hair loss on a cellular level.

Medications that prevent DHT hair loss have formulas to either prevent the conversion of testosterone to DHT, inhibiting DHT's ability to bind to cellular receptor sites, or increase the breakdown and excretion of DHT. Once DHT levels in the scalp are decreased, the cycle of hair loss experienced by dormant follicles is corrected, allowing new hair re-growth to resume.

Vitamin B6 and Zinc

Azelaic acid is a naturally occurring dicarboxylic acid found in whole grain cereals, rye, barley, and animal products. It is FDA-approved as a topical preparation for the treatment of acne and it is effective against a number of other skin conditions when applied topically. There is strong scientific evidence that azelaic acid and zinc are potent inhibitors of 5-alpha-reductase. When azelaic acid, Vitamin B6, and zinc sulfate were added together at low concentrations, 90 percent inhibition of 5-alpha-reductase activity was obtained. The synergistic activity of these compounds against 5-alpha-reductase makes this combination potentially a very effective hair growth formula for treatment of male-pattern baldness.

A Hair Growth Formula for DHT Hair Loss

There are some natural hair growth formulas that combine GLA, ALA, linoleic acid, azelaic acid, Vitamin B6, zinc sulfate, and saw palmetto extracts. By decreasing the DHT levels, hair follicles can grow and thicken naturally, leading to a fuller, healthier scalp without the side effects associated with synthetic medications.

Available topical treatments (e.g., Rogaine®) Minoxidil can stimulate some degree of hair growth in individuals, but by themselves they cannot always produce full healthy hair re-growth and cosmetic benefits. Combination therapy that combines anti-androgens, autoimmune system protective agents, oxygen free-radical inhibitors, and other hair-growth stimulators to halt hair loss and generate hair re-growth can offer better benefits than using Minoxidil alone.

Minoxidil as a Hair Loss Treatment

Minnoxidil is an FDA-approved hair loss medication for re-growth of lost hair both for men and women. Originally used to treat high blood pressure, Minoxidil is now widely used as a topical solution applied twice daily to treat pattern baldness.

It may improve hair growth in 25 percent and slow hair loss in 90 percent of users. How Minoxidil acts is unclear, but when effective, Minoxidil appears to prolong the growing phase in the hair growth cycle, enlarge follicles, and cause dormant follicles to grow. Minoxidil may take 4 months or longer to produce results. Treatment is relatively expensive and must be continued indefinitely. When Minoxidil is stopped, re-grown hair falls out. Newly grown hair may not be as long or thick as normal hair. It can be lighter, like baby hair, and grows mostly on the top of the head, not at the hairline. Minoxidil is more effective in young men and men with recent-onset hair loss. Skin irritation is the most commonly reported side effect. Dizziness and increased heart rate have also been reported, but rarely.

9 | When Should You See a Doctor?

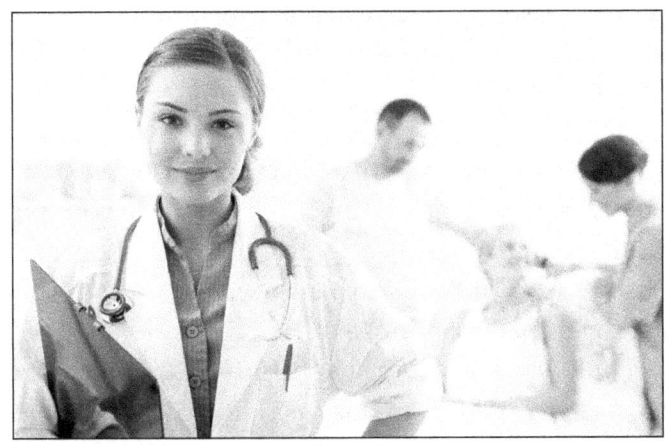

Many doctors don't specialize in hair loss, so seeing doctors in different specialties may actually help you get a better, more accurate diagnosis. There are various conditions of hair loss that might be better served by seeing one more than the other. Perhaps a dermatologist would be better suited to determine if the cause was an infectious scalp condition such as ringworm or scarring alopecia, and an endocrinologist may be better at diagnosing hormone-related hair loss. The truth is that any doctor — whether endocrinologist, dermatologist, or general practitioner — with a strong interest in and knowledge of hair loss can make a proper diagnosis and work with you on the treatment they think will produce the best results. The operative words here are "interest and knowledge."

Try to find a doctor that seems to care about women's hair loss, and understands the emotional devastation it causes. I don't want my doctor to dismiss my hair loss, and I don't want him/her to tell me, "It's no big deal." It *is* a big deal and if your doctor makes you feel uncomfortable in any way, then he/she is not for you. If possible, try to speak with the doctor by phone. Believe it or not, some doctors will talk to you on the phone first. If the rules of the office don't permit this, then try to ask as many questions as possible of the receptionist, such as:

- Does Dr. X see a lot of women for hair loss?
- Does he order blood work?
- What does he usually prescribe for treatment?

The reality of that last question is that there is no "usual treatment." Every woman is different, and hopefully the receptionist will you something to that effect. I don't want to see a doctor that prescribes Rogaine as his/her first line of defense even before making a proper diagnosis with blood work or any other necessary tests. I firmly believe you should not be walking out with a bottle of Rogaine the first day of your appointment. Sure, the doctor can probably tell if your hair is experiencing miniaturization, but what about the blood work to determine the causes? Rogaine may be the right treatment for you, but I'd like to know why.

Trying to figure out exactly what is causing your hair loss is going to require a little detective work on the part of your physician. Several lab tests are going to need to be ordered to start the process. Hopefully, you don't have to bring a list to the doctor's office. He/she should know already. I get concerned when women have to bring to their doctor a list of tests that should be ordered. My feeling is that if they don't know what to order, then how are they going to be able to accurately read the results? But ... a good doctor is a good doctor, and if you have one that really cares and takes a strong interest in your hair loss with willingness to work with you in finding the cause, then great.

Symptom	Diagnosis	Recommended Care
Is your hair falling out in patches?	If hair loss is sudden rather than gradual	See your doctor
Are these patches red, itchy or oily?	This type of hair loss can be caused by SEBORRHEA, PLANUS, or RINGWORM	See your doctor
Are these patches red, itchy or oily?	Small, coin-sized bald areas may be from ALOPECIA AREATA, an autoimmune disease that causes temporary hair loss.	See your doctor
If you notice hair shedding in large amounts while combing or brushing	Many health conditions have a side effect of hair loss and the hair loss may serve as a signal that the body is out of balance.	See your doctor
8-12 weeks after starting a new medication you notice more hair loss than usual	Many medications have a side effect of hair loss.	See your doctor. Discuss your options, there may be an alternate option that will address your health concerns that may not have a side effect of hair loss

Rash, scaliness, or any change in the skin on the scalp with hair loss	Conditions of the scalp can create an unhealthy environment for hair to thrive	See your doctor
Redness Swelling Tenderness or heat Discharge of pus	Scalp inflammation could be a bacterial infection and should be addressed immediately by a medical professional.	See your doctor

So, what exactly is the difference between an endocrinologist and dermatologist?

Endocrinologist: The clinical specialty of endocrinology focuses primarily on the endocrine organs, meaning the organs whose primary function is hormone secretion. These organs include pituitary, thyroid, adrenals, ovaries, testes, and pancreas. An endocrinologist is a doctor who specializes in treating disorders of the endocrine system and who is trained to diagnose and treat hormone problems by helping to restore the normal balance of hormones to your system.

Dermatologist: A dermatologist is a doctor who specializes in the diagnosis and treatment of problems related to the skin, its structure, functions, and diseases, as well as its appendages (nails, hair, sweat glands). The longer definition (as defined by wikipedia): Dermatologists are physicians (Medical Doctors, M.D.) or Doctors of Osteopathy (D.O.) specializing in the diagnosis and treatment of diseases and tumors of the skin and its appendages. There are medical and surgical sides to the specialty. Dermatologic surgeons practice skin cancer surgery (including Mohs' micrographic surgery), laser surgery, photodynamic therapy (PDT), and cosmetic procedures using botulinum toxin (Botox), soft tissue fillers, sclerotherapy, and liposuction.

10

Don't Forget Your Scalp

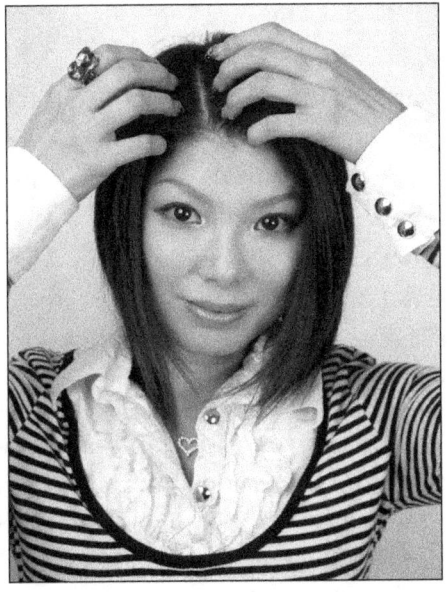

Flakes can be so embarrassing. Let's understand the causes and the cure.

Flaky or itchy scalp produces tiny white pieces of dead skin that flake off the scalp and are usually first noticed on the shoulders. This condition can often be confused with dandruff, but the two are not related. Sometimes the scalp is red or itchy and feels tense. The hair has a dull appearance.

What Causes Flaky Scalp?

- stress
- insufficient rinsing of shampoo
- lack of natural scalp sebum
- using a harsh shampoo
- vitamin imbalance
- pollution
- air-conditioning
- central heating

Dandruff

Dandruff particles are visible flakes of skin that have been continuously shedding from the scalp. It is normal to shed some dead skin flakes, as the skin is constantly renewing itself. The new cells form in the lower layers. They are gradually pushed to the surface as more new cells form beneath them. By the time they reach the surface, the cells have become flat and overlap each other like roof tiles. By then, these cells are dead and are shed from the surface all the time. They are so small that we do not notice this is happening.

With dandruff, this whole process of skin renewal (or skin turnover) speeds up, so a greater number of dead cells are being shed. Also, the cells are shed in clumps, which are big enough to be seen with the naked eye as embarrassing flakes, especially when they land on dark clothing. The scalp may also feel slightly itchy.

Dandruff is very common. It affects more than 50 percent of the population of the USA —so it is more common to have dandruff than not! It can occur at any age, but is most likely in the early 20s.

Causes of Dandruff

Surprisingly, dandruff is a bit of an enigma. About 25 years ago, dermatologists started to blame a tiny fungus, the *Malassezia* yeast, on the scalp. Everyone has some *Malassezia* yeast on their skin, particularly in the greasy areas such as the scalp and upper back. It feeds on the natural grease of the skin, from which it produces oleic acid. The oleic acid triggers increased turnover of skin cells, resulting in dandruff. So, getting rid of the yeast should improve the dandruff.

Hormones may also be involved, because dandruff usually starts after puberty and is more common in men than women. For unknown reasons, people with some illnesses, such as Parkinson's disease, are more likely to have dandruff.

Common beliefs about dandruff — true or false?

- **Dandruff is due to dryness of the skin**
  - » False. Dandruff is caused by a rapid turnover of cells, so more dead cells are shed from the surface. In fact, dandruff occurs in areas where the oil glands of the skin are most active, and the skin is not usually dry.

- **Dandruff is more common in males than in females**
  - » True. Probably because the oil glands are affected by hormones.

- **Dandruff is affected by the weather**
  - » Probably true. Sunlight inhibits the growth of the *Malassezia* yeast.

- **Dandruff results from poor hygiene**
  - » False. Dandruff is caused by rapid turnover of skin cells, probably as a reaction to the *Malassezia* yeast. However, dandruff sufferers do not have more of the yeast than other people —they are just more sensitive to it.

- **Dandruff is contagious**
  - » False. You can not "catch" dandruff from someone else, such as by using his/her brush or comb.

- **Wearing a hat worsens dandruff**
  - » Possibly true. *Pityrosporum* ovale yeasts thrive best when

protected from sunlight. Also, wearing a hat prevents sweat from evaporating, and this may encourage the yeast.

Getting rid of dandruff

- Hair gels and other hair products can irritate the scalp in some people. For a while, try doing without whatever you have been using, or change to a different product.

- Do not scratch your scalp. When you shampoo, massage your scalp without scratching. Scientists have looked at hair from dandruff sufferers who scratch, using an electron microscope that magnifies 400 times. They could see fingernail marks, damaging the hair at its root.

- If your dandruff is mild, try shampooing your hair twice a week using any shampoo labeled "frequent use, for dry hair" (not an ordinary "anti-dandruff" shampoo). This will remove the flakes that are being shed, and the moisturizer in the shampoo will protect the scalp.

- Avoid dyeing your hair (unless you absolutely must). We all have bacteria on our scalp, some of which are beneficial. These "good" bacteria prevent dandruff yeast, and hair dyes reduce their numbers.

- If you want to try a natural remedy, boil four heaped table-spoons of dried thyme in half a liter of water (just under a pint) for 10 minutes. Let it cool and strain it through a sieve into a jar. Massage some of the liquid onto your scalp three times a week. Do not rinse it out.

- Look for a shampoo containing tea tree oil. Research from Australia (published in the *Journal of the American Academy of Dermatology* in 2002) showed that a 5 percent tea tree oil shampoo improved dandruff by 41 percent, which means that, although it did not get rid of the dandruff completely, there was a noticeable improvement.

- For more severe dandruff, you need to deal with the yeast. This means looking carefully at the small print on the anti-dandruff shampoo in your local pharmacy. You could start by trying a shampoo containing selenium sulfide, which has an anti-yeast effect. Wet your hair, rub the shampoo onto your scalp, and rinse off. Repeat, leaving the shampoo for 3 – 5 minutes before rinsing off. Do not use selenium sulfide within 48 hours of applying a hair colorant or a perm lotion. Some shampoos contain zinc pyrithione, another anti-yeast chemical.

- The most effective treatment is an anti-yeast shampoo containing ketoconazole which, in some countries, you can buy from a pharmacist without a doctor's prescription. Wet your hair, rub the shampoo onto your scalp, and rinse off. Repeat, leaving the shampoo for 3 – 5 minutes before rinsing off. Use it twice a week for 2 – 4 weeks to clear the dandruff, and then once every 2 weeks, using a normal shampoo in between times.

- Anti-dandruff conditioners are also available.

When should you see a doctor about dandruff?

- You should certainly see your family doctor if your scalp is red and itchy — or if the skin is flaky around the eyebrows, around the nose or behind the ears — because this suggests you have the more severe form called seborrheic dermatitis (seborrheic eczema). You should also see your doctor if the dandruff is very lumpy or patchy, or if you have scaly skin elsewhere, because it could be a skin disorder, such as psoriasis.

When it's more than a few flakes

Eczema?

Eczema is a general term for many types of skin inflammation, also known as dermatitis. The most common form of eczema is atopic dermatitis (some people use these two terms interchangeably). However, there are many different forms of eczema.

Eczema can affect people of any age, although the condition is most common in infants, and about 85 percent of people have an onset prior to 5 years of age. Eczema will permanently resolve by age 3 in about half of affected infants. In others, the condition tends to recur throughout life. People with eczema often have a family history of the condition or a family history of other allergic conditions, such as asthma or hay fever. Up to 20 percent of children and 1-2 percent of adults are believed to have eczema. Eczema is slightly more common in girls than in boys. It occurs in people of all races.

Eczema is not contagious, but since it is believed to be at least partially inherited, it is not uncommon to find members of the same family affected.

What are the causes of eczema?

Doctors do not know the exact cause of eczema, but a defect of the skin that impairs its function as a barrier, possibly combined with an abnormal function of the immune system, is believed to be important factors. Studies have shown that in people with atopic dermatitis, there are gene defects that lead to abnormalities in certain proteins that are important in maintaining the barrier of normal skin.

Substances that come in contact with the skin, such as soaps, cosmetics, clothing, detergents, jewelry, or sweat, can trigger some forms of eczema. Environmental allergens (substances that cause allergic reactions) may also cause outbreaks of eczema. Changes in temperature or humidity, or even psychological stress, can lead to outbreaks of eczema in some people.

What are the symptoms of eczema?

Eczema most commonly causes dry, reddened skin that itches or burns, although the appearance of eczema varies from person to person and varies according to the specific type of eczema. Intense itching is generally the first symptom in most people with eczema. Sometimes, eczema may lead to blisters and oozing lesions, but eczema can also result in dry and scaly skin. Repeated scratching may lead to thickened, crusty skin.

While any region of the body may be affected by eczema, in children and adults, eczema typically occurs on the face, neck, and the insides of the elbows, knees, and ankles. In infants, eczema typically occurs on the forehead, cheeks, forearms, legs, scalp, and neck.

Eczema can sometimes occur as a brief reaction that leads to symptoms for only a few hours or days, but in other cases, the symptoms persist over a longer time and are referred to as chronic dermatitis.

Food limitation:

To avoid further aggravating your eczema, you need to eliminate certain foods, which could cause some allergic reaction. The following types of food might cause an allergy: seafood, eggs, milk, mango, citrus, peanuts, and tomato.

Scalp Psoriasis May Cause Some Hair Loss

When psoriasis develops on the scalp, hair loss sometimes follows. What may surprise most people is that the root cause of this hair loss is not the psoriasis. Understanding why hair loss occurs and how to manage scalp psoriasis can help.

- **Scales removed too forcefully**. When scalp psoriasis is severe, very thick scales tend to develop. Forcefully removing these scales often loosens the hair as well as the scales.

- **Frequent scratching**. Psoriasis can be incredibly itchy, but frequently scratching the scalp can pull on the hair. Repetitive pulling can lead to a type of hair loss called *traction alopecia*.

- **Psoriasis treatment too harsh**. Sometimes the psoriasis treatment causes the hair loss. Certain medications used to treat scalp psoriasis such as salicylic acid can temporarily damage the hair and lead to hair loss. Also, any treatment that is too vigorous or frequently used can break the hairs and cause hair loss. In most cases, hair grows back when the treatment stops.

- **Stress**. Having psoriasis can be stressful. For some people, stress leads to hair loss. Research shows that stress can cause too many hairs to enter the resting (telogen) phase of the hair growth cycle. Hair stays in the resting phase for about 3 months. At the end of this phase, the body sheds all of the hair in the resting phase. When too much hair goes into the resting phase at one time, the body sheds large amounts of hair at once.

Dermatologists' Tips for Controlling Scalp Psoriasis

While it may seem nearly impossible to control the causes of hair loss associated with scalp psoriasis, effectively managing scalp psoriasis can diminish hair loss. Here are tips that dermatologists often give their patients struggling to control scalp psoriasis:

Treatment

- **Remove scales with gentle combing or brushing**. Loosening and removing scales is an essential part of treating scalp psoriasis. The key is to do it gently. Picking at the scales can aggravate the skin and cause psoriasis to flare. Over time, the picking also can cause traction alopecia, a type of hair loss.

- **Treat the scalp, not the hair.** When applying a topical psoriasis medication, including medicated shampoos, be sure the treatment reaches the scalp and does not sit in the hair.

- **If a treatment seems too harsh, talk with a dermatologist.** Skin on the scalp is thick, so treatment for scalp psoriasis may be stronger than the medication applied to other areas. If the medication causes concern, talk with a dermatologist. There are a number of treatments for scalp psoriasis. Rotating treatments can help, as can switching to another treatment.

- **If nothing seems to stop hair loss, consult a dermatologist**. There are many causes of hair loss. The cause of a patient's hair loss may have nothing to do with psoriasis or its treatment. Hereditary thinning or balding, which is the most common cause of hair loss, affects millions. A dermatologist can help determine the root cause of hair loss and recommend treatment options.

Hair Care

- **Try alternating shampoos**. Using a medicated shampoo one day and a non-medicated shampoo the next can help avoid over-drying of the scalp and hair. Be sure to discuss this strategy with a dermatologist before trying it.

- **Use conditioner after every shampoo**. Applying a conditioner after every shampoo can help keep the scalp moist. A non-medicated conditioner also may help reduce the odor left behind by some tar shampoos.

- **Let hair air dry**. Skin affected by psoriasis is extremely dry. Blow-drying can increase the dryness and exacerbate hair loss. Limiting use of blow dryers and styling products helps to reduce the dryness.

- **Discuss hairstyling options with a dermatologist first**. While hair colors, perms, straightening, and hairsprays can boost self-esteem, they also can irritate scalp psoriasis. Sometimes the chemicals damage already fragile hair, leading to hair loss. Before using any of these hair-care products, either test the product on a small area or ask a dermatologist when such a product can be used.

Self-Care

- Keep fingernails short. For many, scratching is inevitable. Short nails can prevent scratching the scalp so hard that it bleeds.

Most people living with psoriasis experience good days when their skin clears and bad days when psoriasis flares. A trigger is usually needed to make psoriasis appear whether it is for the first time or the thirtieth. Common psoriasis triggers are:

- Infection
- Reaction to certain medications
- Skin injury
- Stress
- Weather
- Other (hormones, smoking, heavy alcohol consumption)

Stress

Ask anyone with psoriasis what triggers a flare-up, and stress is likely to top the list. Scientific studies confirm that stress can worsen psoriasis and increase itching. Some people can even trace their first outbreak to a particularly stressful event.

Having psoriasis is, in itself, stressful. When lesions are visible, people may stare and not want to get near. They may ask, "What did you do to your skin?" Even a spouse, parents, children, friends, and co-workers can be visibly uncomfortable. Some people report that a spouse cannot bear to touch them during severe outbreaks. Others say they feel embarrassed by or ashamed of their skin.

When psoriasis develops on the hands and feet, it is often difficult for people to perform daily tasks, such as picking up objects, typing, and walking. This can make holding a job or caring for a child extremely challenging. The itching and pain caused by psoriasis also makes daily life difficult.

Treating psoriasis can add to the stress. Some treatments are time-consuming. Broadband phototherapy requires three to five visits per week to a clinic, and narrowband requires two to three. Topical medications can be time-consuming to apply. After spending time and money to treat the psoriasis, a person may find the treatment ineffective. Potential side effects deter some people from opting for systemic medications, such as methotrexate and cyclosporine. The cost of treating psoriasis adds stress to many people's lives. Some living with psoriasis find that they cannot afford to pay for the newer treatments such as the biologics.

When the everyday stress of living with psoriasis is compounded by a stressful event at work, a personal crisis, or an especially hectic time, such as the holidays, the stress can feel overwhelming.

People may try to alleviate stress with an herbal or natural over-the-counter remedy. However, some food supplements and herbal remedies interact negatively with prescription medications. People also turn to alcohol and other drugs to reduce stress. Research shows that this actually increases stress.

Dermatologists recommend that their patients tell them if they feel overwhelming stress. There are many healthy ways to relieve stress. Many patients find that psychological counseling or joining a support group effectively reduces stress. Your dermatologist may be able to help you find a therapist or a support group. Some patients prefer to adopt a popular relaxation technique such as meditation. Exercise also can help reduce stress.

Psoriasis is a chronic, non-contagious skin disease characterized by red scaly patches. It may cause lesions, patches, or papules on the surface of the skin and may occur anywhere on the body. The most common causes are immune system disorder and heredity.

Diet restriction

To avoid further aggravating your psoriasis, you need to eliminate certain foods, which might generate toxins inside your body. These foods include: alcohol, coffee, spicy food, shellfish, tropical fruit (mango, pineapple), and red meats.

Weather

Winter tends to be the most challenging season for people living with psoriasis. Numerous studies indicate cold weather is a common trigger for many people and that hot and sunny climates appear to clear the skin.

Cold winter weather is dry, and indoor heat robs the skin of needed moisture. This usually worsens psoriasis. Psoriasis can become even more severe when the stress of the holidays and winter illnesses combine to compromise immune systems

11

Creamy Crack and Other Cosmetic Addictions

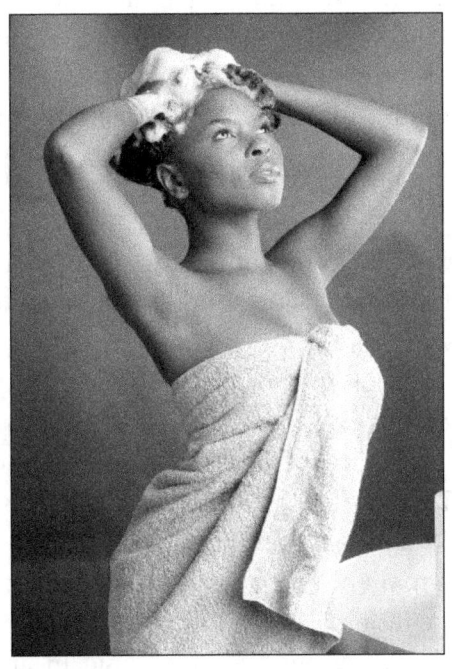

Chemical Abuse is a major cause of damaged hair. When products like relaxers and hair color are easily accessible, anyone can buy them and use them. When chemicals aren't used properly, damaged hair is on the way. It can be especially difficult to apply a relaxer only to your hair's new growth, which is why paying a professional to do this is highly recommended. Overlapping relaxers on previously re-laxed hair makes it weaker and will eventually lead to breakage.

Permanent color, bleaching products, or highlights on hair can be damaging because a percentage of hair's protein is lost during the process, automatically rendering it weaker. Blond hair color on bone-straight relaxed tresses is just asking for trouble. The lifting and depositing process on hair that's already chemically processed can be risky even when done by an experienced beauty professional. Treating double-processed hair is challenging at best.

Over-processing the hair is the most common cause of physical hair damage by far. Perming, straightening, bleaching, and dyeing the hair all involve quite harsh chemicals that can significantly affect the in-tegrity and strength of hair. Using chemical applications improperly can lead to irreversible damage to the hair. The more hair fiber is damaged by these processes, the weaker it will be and the more likely to break off.

The hair cuticle is a very strong outer sleeve of the hair strand. The cuti-cle helps protect the softer inside structure of the cortex from damage. The overlapping scales of the cuticle become damaged when they are exposed to too much processing. For perms, relaxers, straighteners, bleaches, and dyes to work, the cuticle has to be opened up so that other chemicals can get to the hair cortex and rearrange the chemical bonds in the hair structure, as occurs with perms and straighten-ers. The same rule applies when you remove or add hair pigment, as occurs with permanent hair color, bleaching, and highlighting. If manufacturers' directions are not followed and the chemicals used to open the cuticle are applied for too long, in an unsuitably high concentration, or too frequently, the cuticle may be damaged beyond repair. When this happens, the softer cortex is exposed to the environ-ment. The cortex does not have the same properties of the cuticle; it has a rough surface, so at this stage the hair can look dull, "dry," and frizzy. Chemicals in shampoos, in the water, and in air pollution, com-bined with UV light exposure, can all contribute to further damage and weakening of the hair cortex. Eventually, the hair may become so weak that it splits or breaks off completely. Usually, this splitting and breakage occurs to old hair — that is, toward the end of the hair fiber. However, if the chemical processing is very severe, it alone can do so much damage to the hair fiber that the fiber at the root is severely weakened. If this happens, the hair may break off at the skin surface. The result is a diffuse "alopecia" (hair loss).

Physical damage to the hair through over-processing is difficult to treat. The best approach is to cut off as much damaged hair as possible, avoid further chemical processing, be gentle with your hair, and wait for new, undamaged hair to grow in. While there are cosmetic treatments to help "glue" damaged hair back together, they work for only a short time and have to be reapplied regularly. The end result is never as good as the original, undamaged hair. The best way to rid yourself of splits is to cut them off.

One chemical process that can cause damage when not done properly is permanent relaxers. The debate is ongoing as a discussion of whether women with excessively curly and kinky hair should relax their hair or not. Sales of home relaxers have totaled $45.6 million (excluding Wal-Mart), according to Mintel, a market research firm, a figure that has held steady in recent years. Though many of us have had some experience with relaxers, not many of us truly know the origin of hair relaxers.

The relaxer was discovered by an African-American named Garrett Augustus Morgan. Morgan was born the seventh of eleven children to former slaves. He is best known for his invention of the automatic traffic signal and gas mask. But, it was around 1910 that he stumbled upon what would become his contribution to the hair care products industry and what would pave the way for several other entrepreneurs and manufacturers over the next hundred years.

While working in a sewing machine repair shop attempting to invent a new lubricating liquid for the machine needle, it is widely believed that Morgan wiped his hands on a wool cloth. He returned the next day and found the woolly texture of the cloth had "smoothed out."

Morgan set out to find how the liquid chemical had changed the texture as it had. He experimented on an Airedale dog, known for their curly-textured hair. The effect was successfully duplicated.

Morgan then tried his lubricating liquid invention on himself. He called it a "hair refining cream," and thus patented the first chemical hair straightener. Morgan founded a personal grooming products company which included hair dyeing ointments, curved-tooth pressing combs, shampoo, hair-pressing gloss, and the one that started it all: the "G.A. Morgan's Hair Refiner Cream" (advertised to "Positively Straighten Hair in 15 Minutes").

Today, we discuss social, cultural, and political aspects of relaxing or not relaxing one's hair. Consider the bigger question of long-term aftereffects if the act is not performed correctly: hair breakage, hair thinning, and lack of hair growth; scalp irritation, scalp damage, and hair loss. These are just some of the complaints from many who experience problems due to the *misuse* of chemical hair relaxers. In fact, the FDA lists hair straighteners and hair dyes among its top consumer complaint areas. Because of the fragile nature of highly textured hair, the use of any chemical process should always be done with caution and patience. Following manufacturer's directions is a must.

Do You Need Creamy Crack Rehab?

It seems that more women want a hair make-over from chemically relaxed to natural, and it has become a frequently asked question I encounter from women of all ages.

"How can you transition out of the relaxer to natural hair without extreme breakage?"

A common fear is that if you don't continue to have your hair relaxed, all of your relaxed hair will break off — thus the concept of "Creamy Crack." Unfortunately, breakage does happen, in many cases. This occurs as new un-relaxed hair grows past the normal re-touch time. The new hair is strong and often coarse. The point at which the new strong hair joins with the previously relaxed hair which has been straightened and weakened by the chemical relaxer becomes the survival of the fittest. The weaker, relaxed hair cannot win because these two textures cannot co-exist on one strand and the weak hair breaks away. The process of growing an entirely new head of hair that you can style and enjoy requires patience and commitment. I've been through the process of growing out of a relaxer, and it takes patience and a plan. Let's not forget the commitment.

Option 1

- Step 1: Grow it out.
    - » This step requires a lot of patience, but sometimes it is the only way to transition from relaxed hair back to your natural hair. Hair grows at a length of ¼ – ½ inch per month, so it may take 9 months to 2 years or more to truly grow out your relaxed hair. Of course, that will depend on how you care for your hair and how much length will make you feel comfortable.

- Step 2: Trim Gradually
    - » The easiest rule of thumb is growing an inch and then cutting an inch. Remember, condition regularly and take care and patience with your hair. It is very fragile when you have both relaxed and natural texture on one strand. Hair will tend to break off at the point where the 2 textures meet, with the weaker part of the strand, the relaxed part, breaking off.

- Step 3: Condition — Condition — Condition
    - » It is important that you never skip this step. Keeping hair balanced between strength from proteins and softened with moisturizers will be key to a healthy transition.

- Step 4: Set and Go
    - » Wear textured styles — straw sets, rod set styles, and two-strand twisted styles, which will keep hair healthy and

allow the new texture to marry with the relaxed hair with minimal damage.

Option 2

The Big Chop: Cutting all (or most) of the relaxed hair and starting fresh is one of the fastest ways to go from relaxed hair to natural hair.

Option 3

Style your hair in cornrows, braids, extensions, or wigs until the natural hair grows out. This will allow you to look stylish while simultaneously transitioning from relaxed hair to your natural hair. The key here is make sure braids or extensions are not too tight and are conditioned regularly.

During the process, you may find yourself doing any or all of the options above. Just be patient and don't give up. Consult with a professional who can ease you through your journey.

Is All Hair the Same?

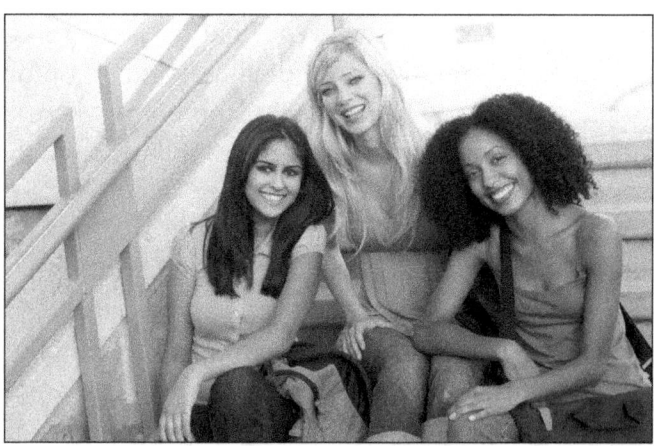

All hair is the same in its makeup. Yes, straight, wavy, curly, or kinky, it's all the same. Every strand of hair is a combination of carbon, hydrogen, nitrogen, oxygen, and sulphur. The major difference in hair is the shape. So girls, those of us with curly and kinky hair have the biggest challenge. The tighter the curl pattern in your hair, the more fragile your hair tends to be. Highly textured hair has many challenges, and eighty percent of all African-American hair is characterized as tight or excessively curly. It has been determined that there are approximately six to eight levels of curl texture, and problems begin with improper manipulation of the twists and turns in the tightly curled hair shaft. Stress accumulates at the twists of tightly curled hair; this stress point is fragile and is a weak spot where elasticity naturally diminishes. Where stress has accumulated, combing, brushing, styling and chemical processes can be more damaging to excessively curly hair than straight hair. This hair is extremely fragile and requires gentle handling.

Want to Grow Your Hair?

Just Love Your Hair

As a third-generation beauty professional, one thing has not changed over the generations: healthy hair is a timeless classic. Trends will come and go, but never trade the health of your hair for a trendy style. I'm not one to micromanage, but when it comes to hair, I'm guilty. Manage the details and be very particular about what goes on with your hair and who handles your hair. When possible, seek out the best hair care professional and develop an ongoing relationship of communication and trust. It's important to have a professional who knows your hair and can proactively address subtle or drastic changes. It doesn't seem fair, but you can take great care of your hair and make one mistake with color, relaxers, or heat and it can ruin your hair in one day. It can take years to get your hair back to a good place, so love your hair and micromanage your hair care.

The truth is, we all have had that moment when we look in the mirror after combing, brushing, spraying, pushing, and pulling, and say the words out loud: "I Hate My Hair!" Even though you don't really mean it, at that moment, you felt it. We have such an involved love/hate affair with our hair. Our hair can become our obsession, especially when hair is less than perfect.

With all the obsessing, you must remember to love your hair, and treat it gently. Your face is the picture and your hair is the frame. Your hair is a delicate fiber; treat it as gently as possible. Just as you provide the gentlest treatment for your finest washables, you should take the same approach with your hair. Treat it like an expensive fine silk blouse, not an old pair of denim cut-offs. Surprisingly, people treat their hair poorly and then wonder why it's damaged. I've come to realize that for many, they just don't realize the damage they inflict with simple, seemingly harmless acts.

Make Hair Grow Faster?

If I had a dollar for every time I've been asked, "What can I buy or do to make my hair grow faster?" I would be a very wealthy woman.

There is no magic formula

Yes, there are lots of things that can maximize your hair growth, but don't imagine that you can go to bed one night with 6 inches of hair and after one week of a magical potion, you'll wake up a week later with 12 inches of your own hair. It's not going to happen unless you get some extensions.

Hair for most people is genetically programmed to grow a maximum of 4-6 inches a year if you can keep it healthy enough to maintain every inch you grow.

Unfortunately, many people aren't aware of the fact that while hair can be extraordinarily resilient, once it has emerged from your scalp it has no facility for renewing itself. It is considered to be dead protein.

The average person has around 150,000 strands of hair on their head and the average rate of growth can range from one eighth up to one-half of an inch per month. This rate of growth can vary based on texture, type, and condition.

By the time the ends of your hair actually grow down to your shoulders, they are approximately two years old.

Think about it. Two years is a long time for hair to be subjected to the daily wear and tear, shampooing, blow drying, flat ironing, curling, brushing, combing, and often repeated chemical processing with relaxers, perms, and hair color. Just imagine what a piece of silk or fine fabric would look like after 2 years of constant handling.

The Wonders of Scalp Massage

Scalp massage, as hair loss prevention, has been used throughout history by many different cultures. Massaging the scalp should be part of every hair loss regime.

One of the most obvious benefits of scalp massage is increased circulation. The scalp is one of the hardest places for blood to flow. The increased blood flow helps to nourish the follicle. The scalp depends on blood flow to bring oxygen and nutrients to the hair follicles.

Tension causes tightness in the scalp, which restricts blood flow and can cause hair loss. Scalp massage restores pliability and relieves tension, helping to create an ideal environment for new hair growth.

Massaging the scalp also helps loosen and remove dead cells and excess sebum on the scalp, which can hinder new hair growth. Scalp massage helps to distribute the hair's natural oils to protect and condition the hair.

The benefits of scalp massage go beyond hair loss prevention. Seventy percent of our nervous system is in the head. Scalp massage activates neural pathways to the brain and stimulates unused brain cells. Besides that, scalp massage feels good! It is nurturing and relaxing to the whole body.

Scalp massage can also include the face and neck. You can perform it yourself or have someone do it for you. Slide your fingertips under your hair and onto your scalp. Use the balls of your fingertips. Use gentle circular motions to stimulate your entire scalp.

12

Strand Strategies for Every Age

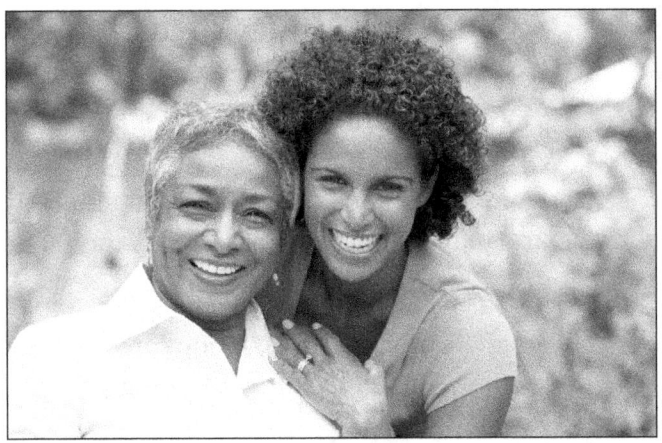

Strand Strategies in Your Twenties

Estrogen, which is a huge driver of hair growth in women, is at peak levels in your twenties. Now is a time to experiment with your hair, but beware of tight ponytails and braided styles that are too tight; too much tension can lead to traction alopecia, which if not treated early can become a permanent condition.

Beware of all the blow drying, curling, straightening, and flat ironing that goes into those complicated styles, which can leave hair dry, brittle, and vulnerable to breakage. Curb damage by always conditioning after shampooing, and using heat appliances only on freshly shampooed hair. When you are using heat tools, opt for ionic dryers and ceramic styling tools, which are gentler on hair. Prep and protect hair with a lightweight thermal protectant spray to guard against damaging heat. Give your hair a rest between heat sessions by setting or wrapping hair. Freshly heat-styled hair can look fabulous and full of body, but there is the underlying danger of overdoing a good thing. When heat is used too often, and especially when hair is chemically relaxed, permanently colored, highlighted, or bleached, the threat of damage is real. Double or even triple that threat for hair that is highly textured.

Strand Strategies in Your Thirties

Thanks to stress and hormonal shifts that kick in around thirty, your hair can start to show signs of thinning and look a little limp. Your best defense is a softly layered cut. Ask for long layers that start at the edge of your outer lip and graduate down from there. Blunt-cutting the back of the hair can give the illusion of fullness and thickness.

Freaking out about your first gray strands? No worries; temporary color can turn gray strands into highlights without any damage. It's like magic, turning that stumbling block into a stepping stone.

This is the time in life where you become so busy with family and career that you have less time for self. Typically, women begin to request and require low- to no-maintenance styles. This is also a time when there's a little more financial stability, and weaves and extensions seem even more appealing. Just be careful, and do not allow braids or extensions to be applied with too much tension, as this can lead to traction alopecia, which can become a permanent condition. Here's a foolproof tip: if it feels too tight for more than 48 hours, it's too tight and you should have it removed.

Strand Strategies in Your Forties and Beyond

Lots of women get a short "sensible" hair cut in their forties. Some may think this to be a practical choice, considering that declining estrogen levels can cause hair to appear thinner, dull, and frizzy. Here's the thing — chopping off your hair can expose parts of your face and neck that had been concealed or at least softened by longer hair. Instead of the big chop, ask your stylist for a cut with movement and texture. For example, you could go for neck- or shoulder-length hair with subtle layers and sideswept bangs. This look can hide a multitude of sins. Bangs are a cheap and easy way to make your look chic and modern. The also accentuate the positive and camouflage the negative. This haircut "cure-all" hides a large forehead, forehead lines, or a receding hairline. At the same time, a soft fringe of hair falling along the side of your face draws attention up to the eyes (the windows of the soul), and deflects scrutiny away from the jaw line, which may be a little saggy or slack.

Lighten up

Your twenty-something shade won't work when you're 50. Extremely dark hair can look hard and fake next to mature skin. A change from black or espresso brown to a softer shade, like maple or chestnut, can erase years. Some women choose semi-permanent color, which covers some gray but not all. Although it shampoos out in about six weeks, it looks more natural and dimensional than a flat, permanent color.

Gray Hair

Attitude makes it work. Lots of women look fabulous with their natural gray hair. To keep it fresh, gray hair can require a little packaging, or the look can slip from great to granny. Haircut, makeup, and clothes need to be in sync and of-the-minute. Stay in shape and maintain a lively body language. You're only as old as you feel, but remember, we live in a very visual world and looks do matter.

Going Gray?

The aging process —

At some stage in our lives, both men and women will experience the onset of gray hair. Contrary to popular belief, gray hair is not always related to age. Gray hair can occur as young as in our teens and range into our late 50s and even older.

Some people start to gray in their early 20s or 30s; this is called premature graying. Their gray hair may look the same when they are older as it did in their 20s or 30s. Other people do not become gray until they are in their 50s or later.

When there is more salt than pepper in your hair, it is a constant reminder that you are no longer young. This reality can be very upsetting. Reactions vary. Should you decide to concentrate on the salt, accept the inevitable, and relegate yourself to being a spectator in life, then no particular action is necessary. However, if the pepper side calls to you, then aggressive steps are needed to retain a high performance.

Everybody is different, but the pigment of our hair is generated in the same way.

Initially, hair is white. The cells in our hair follicles called "melanocytes" generate pigments the main one being melanin. This gives our hair its "color."

In general, the more melanin present, the darker the hair color; the less melanin, the lighter the hair color.

When these melanocytes stop producing the pigment, the result is a transparent hair. The transparent hair against your healthier darker hair gives the appearance of gray hair. In reality the hair is not gray, but transparent. Harvard scientists propose that a failure of melanocyte stem cells (MSC) to maintain the production of melanocytes could cause the graying of hair.

The main reason for our hair turning grey is heredity.

If your mom or dad started going gray at a young age, then the chances are you may also suffer from premature gray hair. This is not always the case. Age does play a large part in the graying process. The pigment in the hair shaft is generated from cells at the base of the root of the hair and as we get older these cells start producing less pigment until there is no pigment at all in the hair and we end up with the transparent hair.

Gray Hair Facts

Pluck one gray hair and two more will grow back — completely false.

- Gray hair can be harder to color, as it is more resistant to hair color or hair dye due to a decreased amount of melanin.
- Gray hair can be the result of a medical condition. If you are deficient in B12 or suffer from a thyroid imbalance it can also cause your hair to go gray.
- When your hair is half white and half colored, it's called "salt and pepper."
- Smokers are 4 times more likely to have gray hair than nonsmokers, and smoking has been conclusively linked to accelerated hair loss.

Can hair turn gray overnight?

Hair turns gray slowly over time. As you get older, the production of your color pigment slows down and gray hair begins to appear.

Can you get grey hair from a fright or psychological shock or trauma?

Studies have shown that if this does happen, then it's typically due to alopecia areata. What happens here is that the thicker, darker hair stops growing before it affects the growth of gray hairs, giving the impression of gray hair overnight.

In some cases, gray hair may instead be caused by a deficiency of B12 or a thyroid imbalance.

Gray hair is more noticeable in people with darker hair because it stands out, but people with naturally lighter hair are just as likely to go gray.

Your chance of going gray increases 10 – 20 percent every decade after you turn 30.

The Importance of Drinking Water

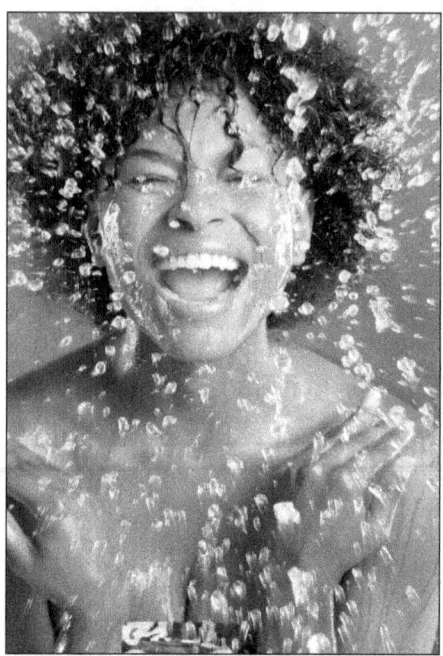

It is amazing to me that I meet so many people who say they don't drink water! What? Water is essential for any living thing.

The benefits of drinking water are extraordinary. Pure drinking water is the most important nutrient of all. Yet the health benefits of drinking water are often ignored.

Every cell and system in your body relies on water to operate properly. Although you could live for over a month without food, you can go for only about 3 days without water.

The importance of drinking water and getting water benefits is essential to life — second only to oxygen. It's a major component of your skin, tissues, cells, and all of your organs.

Water is necessary to process and absorb all the nutrients from the foods you eat. It circulates through your blood and lymphatic system, carrying oxygen and essential nutrients to your cells. It also flushes out toxins and waste through urine and sweat.

Consistent lack of enough water (chronic dehydration) can cause constipation problems, hypertension, asthma, allergies, migraine headaches, and many other health problems. Every single part of you and your functioning is dependent on water.

For example:

- Your hair is 25 percent water
- Your muscles are about 75 percent water.
- The blood in your veins is 83 percent water.
- Your bones are approximately 23 percent water.
- Your trillions of cells are 64-91 percent water.
- And the brain in your head is 78 percent water.
- Your body is around 66 percent water.

Health Benefits of Drinking Water

As you can see, your very survival is dependent on clean water.

Looking at the many benefits of drinking water, you realize that pure, uncontaminated water could be considered a virtual fountain of youth wonder drug. Taken in optimum doses — about 8 glasses a day — you could produce the following miraculous results:

- Reduce your risk of heart attack.
- Decrease headaches and dizziness.
- Have healthier, younger-looking skin.
- Burn fat, build muscle, and lose weight.
- Improve both digestion and elimination.
- Increase mental clarity and performance.
- Flush toxins from your body more efficiently.
- Lubricate and reduce pain in joints and muscles.
- Reduce your risk of disease and infection, and feel well.
- Increase energy, alertness, and physical performance.

Good hydration also greatly decreases your need for taking medications. Plus, great additional benefits of drinking water are that it's cheap, calorie-free, and very convenient.

Even if you take the best possible care of your hair, your hair still goes through a natural aging process, which can also impact the growing cycle of your hair.

Drink 8 to 10 glasses (8-ounce servings) of water a day to get gleaming healthy tresses. Water makes up approximately one-fourth of the weight of a strand of hair, and when hair has the proper amount of water, it will respond by being supple and shiny. Water is essential for proper hair growth. Be sure to get plenty of that H2O for growing healthy hair that is soft, supple, and lush.

The human body is generally composed of approximately 60-80 percent water. When deprived of adequate water to sustain cell health and reproduction, the body becomes dehydrated, which directly impacts hair growth.

You can be sucking down a fistful of hair vitamins and related hair growth supplements, but if you are not downing enough H2O to meet your body's daily minimal levels, your cells that drive hair growth will not even reproduce and your hair will become parched.

On a regular day, the average human body loses 2 to 3 quarts of water. While water is lost through sweat, urine, and other waste removal, it is also lost in a number of other ways. Human skin has a high concentration of water, which is constantly evaporating in tiny airborne droplets.

Quick tips for Fabulous Hair

Brush with care: it's a myth that we should brush hair 100 times daily. Excessive brushing can be really bad for your hair. If you are too rough in brushing or repeatedly brush the same area, it can lead to breakage and split ends. Brush your hair only as much as you really need to.

Tips for shiny hair:

- Eat plenty of iron-packed foods or take iron supplements. Iron is a good source of nutrients that will give you healthy skin and shiny hair.

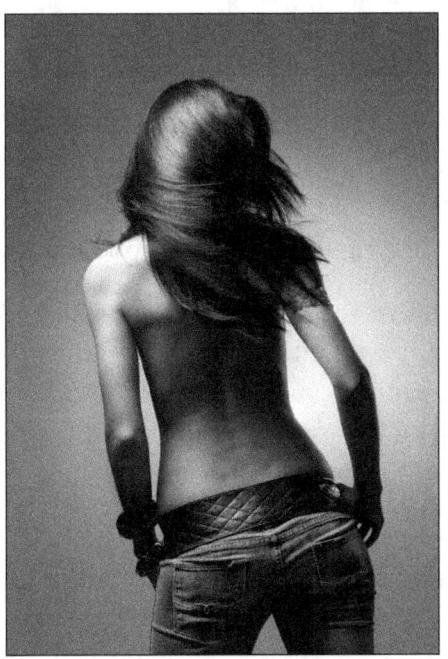

- Vitamin E should be the epitome of shine. Vitamin E has special agents that create a silky, shiny effect for your hair. You can take a supplement or use a product-based gel, shampoo, or conditioner.

- Condition your hair weekly. To get the best results, use a deep conditioner.

- Use hot oil treatments to create great shine.

- Moisturizing shampoos and deep penetrating conditioners are ideal when you are trying to get shiny hair. They help fill empty spaces in the hair shaft and seal in shine.

Do not overdo the use of a curling iron or the flat iron. Your hair will experience heat damage if you use these hairstyling methods too frequently. It is best to not use them any more than twice a week. Also be sure to use a quality heat protectant product to buffer the damage associated with the use of hot tools.

Wet hair is the weakest, so comb gently, starting at the ends to release tangles. Use a leave-in detangling product, to assist in the release of tightness and tangles.

Frizzy hair can be caused by rough treatments, such as too much harsh brushing or pulling the hair into rubber bands.

Dry hair looks dull, feels dry, tangles easily, and is difficult to comb or brush, particularly when it is wet. It is often quite thick at the roots but thinner and sometimes split at the ends. Dry hair can be identified quickly by its dull, lackluster appearance. This is often the result of excessive perming or coloring. However, sometimes it can be because the scalp has fewer oil glands than normal.

Split ends cannot be mended, just temporarily sealed. The only permanent cure is to have your hair trimmed regularly

Hair for All Seasons

Keep Hair Sexy for Summer
The **sun can strip the hair** of its natural oils, and dry heat will only intensify the problem. Just two weeks in the sun without protecting your hair can weaken hair cuticles, with peeling, breaking, and split ends becoming a problem.

A **weakened cuticle leaves hair vulnerable** to dehydration and susceptible to color fading. Sun exposure also encourages free radical activity in the hair shaft. The cells of the hair are damaged, as the free radicals cause premature ageing.

Deep-conditioning treatments are vital, especially before traveling to a hot climate — particularly for chemically treated hair. However, the only way to protect your hair 100 percent from sun damage is to keep it out of the sun. A hat is the best option.

Fine hair: Pack a gentle shampoo and a light leave-in conditioner with UV protection. A sun-protection spray that contains a UV filter will help screen the hair from the sun and seawater if you are planning fun in the sun on a beach. Re-apply the protectant through the hair after each dip in the sea.

Curly hair: Pack a gentle moisturizing shampoo to cleanse your hair, plus a creamy leave-in conditioner to help guard against excess dryness. If you are sunbathing, apply a sun-protection spray or oil that contains a UV filter to reduce sun damage to the hair, and reapply it regularly, just as you would suntan lotion to your face and body. Apply a good nourishing hair mask for beautiful hair.

Frizzy hair tends to be dry anyway, and needs extra care in dry heat. As before, use a sun-protection spray or oil on your hair during the day. Make sure you apply a rich leave-in conditioner with UV protection to your hair each morning before going out in the sun. Apply a hair mask to your hair at least every other day during your holiday. You can leave it on overnight for an intensive treatment if your hair becomes very dry in the heat.

Beware of Winter's Woes

Blood circulation is not as rapid during the colder season. Cold air evaporates the natural moisture of your hair. When that happens, dry hair has almost no defense against everyday damage. Even though your obvious issue is dryness, here's a pro tip: you probably have lost some protein from any chemical treatment, like relaxer, highlights, or full color, and that is the reason your moisture level is low. This means you need to add a balance of protein and moisture to your hair. Use a conditioning combination of protein and moisture.

One of my favorite proteins is soy-based protein mixed with moisturizing agents. You can lock the moisture in by closing the cuticle of your hair with a cool rinse. It is an old but proven technique. Now that you've taken care of your hair, your scalp may also need attention. Scalp produces sebum, oil that is produced naturally. Sebum production can slow down during the winter season, which causes dry and itchy scalp. If you notice these symptoms, treat your scalp with something light and natural, like olive oil, pure coconut oil, or pure shea butter.

Head Gear

Fabrics, such as wool, can create a lot of friction when rubbing against your hair fibers, and even cause breakage. Synthetic fabrics can also draw moisture away from your body. Not wearing a hat is not an option for many, as the winter cold makes it just impossible not to want to keep your head covered somehow. But there are things you can do to prevent your head garments from damaging your hair. For instance, if you wear a wool hat, try lining it with a silk scarf.

Whenever possible, avoid drying your hair with too much direct heat. Also, avoid the over-use of curling irons and flat irons. If you have to use heating tools, consider purchasing a leave-in-conditioner, in addition to the deep conditioner. Purchase natural-based products, like shea butter, that can protect your hair, while you are using heating tools. Keep the use of gel and alcohol-based hairspray to a minimum. If you have to use those products, try to get those that do not have alcohol as an ingredient. Make sure to trim your hair every 6-8 weeks. The longer the hair, the harder it is to protect against winter damage. Your hair is an extension of your body. Drink at least eight glasses of water a day. Do not forget about local beauty salons. Many salons offer treatments to hydrate your hair and scalp.

Don't Get Caught Up

You don't mean to do it, but you put on your coat, scarf, and hat; strap your bag over your shoulder, and your hair gets caught under your coat or the strap of your bag. The tugging and snapping of stands adds up over the winter and can cause quite a bit of breakage.

Beat the Heat: The Inside Story

Heat from buildings may feel good in the winter months, but indoor heat can be very drying to hair and skin. Lots of moisture is removed from the air with dry heat, so check your hair for the drying impact.

Solutions:

- Purchase a humidifier to rehydrate the air
- Increase deep conditioning/hot oil treatments — deep conditioners help heal damaged hair and protect from further damage
- Protect hair
- Protect your ends with natural essential oils like shea butter, olive oil, castor oil, sage oil, peppermint oil
  - » ends take a beating because they are the most aged and abused portion of the hair strand

Get the Look — Create an Illusion

Now that we have covered most of the concerning points of getting and keeping your hair in the best condition possible, let's consider the look you want. Depending on your hair type, texture, and condition, you and your hair stylist should be able to determine the best look to capture your sense of style and the easiest look for you to manage. A naturally healthy hairstyle usually means a cut and style that does not require a lot of products to stay in place or be manageable. Your haircut is the foundation of your hairstyle. If your hairstyle is personalized to your hair type, texture, condition, and lifestyle, you shouldn't have to over-use products or styling tools, or go through excessive wear and tear to get your hair to look great.

It's okay to use styling products and styling tools, but in hairstyling as in life, all things in moderation is the path to balance.

The Cut Creates the Style

Hair reflects our individuality, our fashion statement, and speaks volumes about how we feel about ourselves. When deciding on new and different looks for your hair, ask yourself these questions:

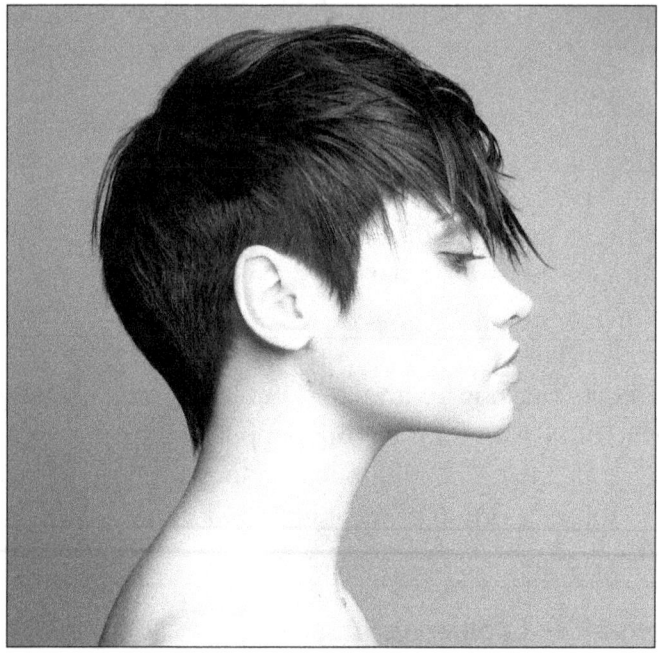

- What are your likes and dislikes about your hair?
- What are you willing to do at home to keep the style looking its best?
- How much time do you have to spend with your hair on a daily basis?
- How often can you return to the salon for deep conditioning and upkeep?

Other considerations are:
- Height
- Weight
- Head shape
- Face shape

Facial features
Balancing your features: the size and shape of your face should be complemented and balanced by the shape of your haircut.

OVAL-Shaped Face

Ovals are considered the ideal face shape. This shape can wear any design with flair! Bobbed, layered, close / full / long or short...just about any style will suit this balanced shape. However, you must take into consideration your facial features. To cancel out narrowness, try tousled curls, lush waves, and dense bangs. The fuller the hair the fuller the face will seem.

SQUARE-Shaped Face

Soften the edges of a square-shaped face by directing soft wavy bangs down over your temples. Long hair should fall to or past shoulders. For a short style, keep hairstyle round and soft with height at the crown. If pulled up, play with wisps of hair around the face. The primary goal here is to soften your angular jaw and forehead. You can essentially erase sharp edges with tapered layers and a flirty fringe.

ROUND-Shaped Face

The goal is to create an oval appearance and lift the face. Keep the sides close to the face and promote height at the crown. Looking for a classic modern style, long subtle layers are perfect for a round face. For short shape, close side wisps soften and flatter the face. Avoid blunt cuts, and keep volume on the top and bottom, not on the sides. Round faces are youthful. Streamlined hair adds sophistication as well.

DIAMOND-Shaped Face

To balance a narrow chin, your best look is a rounded shape with fullness at the bottom. Wide wispy bangs help to create an oval look. The classic look for diamonds is a graduated bob that falls to the chin. Try a wispy design to soften the edges.

PEAR-Shaped Face

Focus on a full crown at top to create symmetry with the wide jaw.

Layered looks, like the classic shag, flatter the pear-shaped face. Cut or style hair short and close at your ear so as to not draw attention to your cheeks.

HEART-Shaped Face

Heart-shaped faces need a softer, curlier style. A chin-length look is perfect. The objective is to create width around your narrow chin. Side-slanted bangs draw attention away from the jaw line. The best look is full /curly / wavy / bouncy. However, you must take into consideration your facial features. The key is to draw attention to your eyes and cheekbones. Brow-grazing fringe and mis-length layers move the focus away from a strong chin.

RECTANGLE-Shaped Face

Go for width and volume. A suitable short style includes the bob design. Long manes in full styles should fall at or above the shoulder. Bangs look great when just touching the brows and help to shorten a long-shaped face. However, you must take into consideration your facial features. Do you want to distract the eye away from a receding hairline? Bangs, for instance, can accent your eyes, while hair off the forehead can balance your nose in profile view.

Find an Extraordinary Salon and Stylist

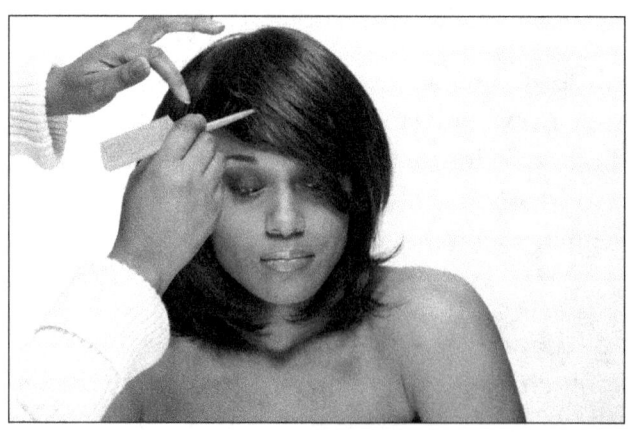

Your new stylist needs to be willing to;

Ask-Listen-Learn

Ask Around

Ask your friends and acquaintances about their stylists. If you see someone on the street who has a hairstyle you admire, don't hesitate to ask for the stylist's name. Most will be flattered and only too happy to tell you.

Pick a salon with a good reputation and ask for a stylist who specializes in your type of hair, or choose one based on what you've heard.

The Consultation

Schedule a consultation and hair analysis. Make sure the stylist asks questions about your hair history, lifestyle, and hairstyling preferences, and inquires about any hair damage, breakage, or hair loss issues. The stylist should also inquire about any health conditions and medications, in that it can have a direct impact on your hair's condition. The stylist should also touch and examine your hair and scalp to determine the condition of both.

A consult is also the ideal time for you to interview the stylist, since you will be hiring her for a very important job. Ask questions about timing and scheduling. Ask about the stylist's hair care philosophy — is it style, health, or a balance of both?

First Contact

Was your phone experience a pleasant one? What is the salon's energy? Observe the sounds, smells, décor, and essence of the salon. Is this a place you would like to spend several hours on a regular basis? Is the salon clean and orderly, or chaotic?

Do Your Homework

Find out as much as you can about that particular stylist, such as how long he or she has been in business and what products he or she prefers.

Discuss the Options

Express your desires for your hair as best you can, and bring pictures of hairstyles you'd love to wear. Be very specific about what you want your hair to do. If you don't know what you want it to do or don't know what it can do, then express that to the stylist. After an informative discussion, your stylist should come up with some ideas. Once you have found the ideal look, the stylist should be able to explain, in an easily understandable way, how he or she will achieve the look.

Throughout the entire service, you should expect the stylist to share information with you, in essence educating you about what is being done and why. At some point during the service the stylist should walk you through the steps to re-create your new look. Once your service is complete, you should find yourself thrilled with your style and the service you received. Professional stylists can be an amazing asset to your life; the key is finding the right fit for you and your hair.

13

Remember: Every Strand Matters

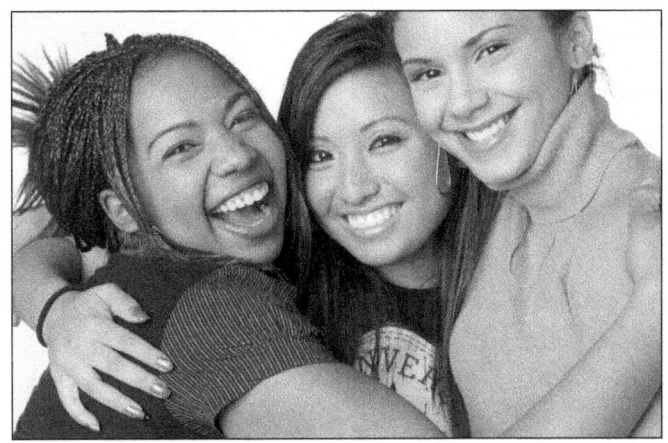

Hair is a very important aspect of our lives, and it definitely connects us to our emotional beauty. You never know how much those strands mean to you until you begin to lose them. We must begin to appreciate the obvious connection between the health and growth of hair and the proper nurture and care of the body, mind, and spirit. When the balance of one of these aspects is disturbed, your hair will show the signs.

The relationship with your hair starts with you. Become an advocate of balance for your life and your hair. Feeling healthy and looking your best brings pleasure and joy. By nurturing your mind, body, spirit, and hair with the information I've shared, you'll be well on your way to healthier hair and a happier you. Approach any future hair challenges with patience, kindness, and love toward your overall self. It's never too late to be proactive. Get to know your hair and your body. Notice subtle changes. Remember to constantly exercise the 3 P's:

- Probe   Investigate changes in your hair — look beyond the surface

- Prescribe   Seek to achieve and maintain balance for your ever-changing hair

- Persist   Stick with a winning program and see it through to success

Begin Today:

Now that you have become familiar with some of the circumstances that can affect your hair, you have the knowledge to move to the next step, whether that means consulting with a professional or taking matters into your own hands. This book was designed to allow you to look at hair condition and growth in a new and more comprehensive way. Yes, we have covered a lot of information, and it may seem overwhelming to figure out where to start. To help you become more proactive, here is a guide to the areas of general concern, which can serve as a conversation starter with your professional practitioner. Begin today to create the head of hair you can fall in love with again.

Be bold and proactive — start with your very own healthy hair analysis:

Gather several strands of hair, about as much as you would put in a straw. Hold it at the very bottom, right where it comes off the scalp, and pull up, out to the ends. Now look to see how many hairs you have in your hand. A straw amount of hair is about 60 hairs. If you're pulling out more than six hairs, (10%) then you're starting to lose hair more rapidly than you should. Test several areas on your head — front, back, top, and sides. If you are consistently pulling hair out during your test, take time to examine the hair strands. Are the strands broken strands, or the full length of your average hair length? Is there a small white bulb attached to the end of the strand? If so, this means this strand has shed from the root. If all or most of the strands in your pull test have a bulb attached, you are shedding hair rapidly and more than likely, there is an internal cause. Refer to chapters 3-7 to identify any possible conditions, medications, or behaviors you might recognize in your life. If you cannot readily identify some possible cause, consider visiting your doctor for a thorough examination, since the condition of the hair is an indicator of the condition of your health.

Be sure to consider the following conditions and/or the medications associated with controlling the condition:

- Allergies
- Stress levels
- Thyroid condition
- Anemia
- Liver disease
- Diabetes
- Acne
- Sleep disorders
- Circulation issues
- Hormonal imbalances
- Abnormal menses
- Kidney disease
- Autoimmune diseases
- Vitamin deficiencies (especially A & D)
- Contraceptives
- Menopausal and post-menopausal conditions
- Genetics (does hair loss run in the family?)

Consider these conditions as well as those outlined in the earlier chapters. Be sure to share your concerns with your physician and your hair professional.

Now let's look at the condition of your existing hair. Hair damage can be caused by a variety of things, including hair color, heat-based styling tools, and improper care. Damaged hair has a distinctive look and feel that's fairly simple to spot if you know what you're looking for. There are several tests you can perform on your locks to determine whether they are damaged. You may be frustrated with your hair and continuously trying new products to correct what you believe to be wrong.

Here are some tests to determine the true condition of your hair:

Sink Test

The sink test measures how porous your locks are. Healthy hair is fairly solid, while damaged hair shafts absorb liquid quickly because they are weak. To perform the sink test, pluck four strands of hair from your head: one from the top, one from the back, and one from each side. Drop the strands of hair in a container of water. If the strands float, they are quite healthy. If they sink, they are damaged. The strands will sink because they have lost the cuticle or outside layer of protection. Without adequate cuticle scales (which equals about 10-15 % of the hair strand) to protect the most important core of the hair strand known as the cortex (which equals 85-90% of the hair strand), the strand cannot survive. When this damaged strand is emerged in water, there is not adequate protection on the outer shell and excess water is absorbed, thus causing the strand to sink.

Tug Test

The tug test measures the elasticity of your hair. Healthy hair is slightly stretchy, while unhealthy hair is brittle and breaks when put under even minor stress. To perform a tug test, dampen a section of your hair. Grip two to three strands between your thumb and forefinger and gently pull on the ends. If it stretches by about one-third of its original length and bounces back when you let go, it's healthy. However, if your hair breaks off, it has suffered some damage to the cortex and is not structurally sound.

Porosity Test

The porosity test determines the condition of your hair cuticle. An undamaged cuticle will feel smooth, but a damaged cuticle with leave hair uneven and coarse. To test your hair's porosity, grasp a section of your hair between your index finger and middle finger. Slide the section of hair through your fingers, going from the tip to the root. If your hair feels rough and uneven, it is damaged. If it feels mostly smooth, the cuticle scales are healthy.

The ultimate in healthy hair is a balance between protein and moisture. Hair is comprised of protein known as keratin. The protein gives hair strength. The moisture provides hair with the flexibility for curl and movement. Most conditioning products available will be either protein or moisture or a combination of the two. The goal of conditioning hair is to find a healthy balance and maintain it. When that balance is achieved, along with a healthy mind, body, and spirit, the hair you desire can be yours.

Remember, Every Strand Matters!

As a hair care expert, I answer questions about hair problems almost every day.

Here is a small sample of some of the most frequently asked questions; perhaps this

can help you find a solution:

Frequently Asked Questions:

Question

My hair is very dry and I have tried everything from less frequent shampooing to moisturizers. What can I do to stop this dryness?

Answer

The key to your dilemma is balance. Hair requires a balance of protein and moisture to maintain its health. Hair is 97% protein and 3%

moisture. If hair lacks the proper protein balance it will be difficult to hold the moisture you are attempting to achieve.

The proper balance of protein allows your hair to hold the moisture — without it, imagine pouring water through a sifter; the holes represent the lack of protein or empty pockets in your hair, and there is no substance in place to hold the moisture. So, try a two-step conditioning regimen: after shampooing, condition with the protein-fortified conditioner of your choice first, to strengthen your hair. Rinse and follow with the moisturizing conditioner of your choice to provide softness and flexibility, and you'll be on your way to a more balanced situation.

Question

My hair is very long and my main worry is that my hair is now thinning, and I'm afraid that I might lose it. Please help.

Answer

There is an alarming number of women who share your concern with thinning. In fact, the latest statistic states that approximately 40 million women suffer thinning and balding hair. This condition can result from a number of contributing factors such as:

- Hormonal imbalance
- Medications
- Medical conditions
- Scalp infections
- Poor nutrition
- Stress
- Heredity
- Excessive tension in hairstyles (tight ponytails/ braids…)

It is recommended that you see a professional to get a proper hair and scalp analysis to determine the cause of your thinning and provide a suggested solution based on your individual needs. Hair loss is progressive and tends to advance if not treated. There are nutritional supplements available that provide a combination of ingredients that will work within the scalp at the hair roots to decrease hair shedding, stimulate hair growth, and improve fullness.

Question

I have color-treated and relaxed hair. Even though my color has been in for 10 months, all of a sudden my hair has started to completely break off between the new growth and the color. I've tried to keep my hair moisturized and away from chemicals and heat, but I still don't know how to stop the breakage.

Answer

Believe it or not your dilemma is common among women who relax and permanently color their hair. Here's the issue: each of these processes permanently alters your hair's structure. The double chemical process causes hair to lose a lot of protein and moisture. Your hair needs the right balance of protein for strength, as well as moisture which gives hair its flexibility and shine.

The double chemical process can weaken the hair strand to the point that any additional chemical treatments, or daily wear and tear, can prove to be too much for the already fragile hair strand and it begins to break.

To slow the breakage, begin a combination of protein and moisture treatments to regain the balance necessary for your strand's health. Additionally, regular trims begin to remove the fragile, breaking hair — you can adopt the theory of grow a healthy inch; trim a fragile damaged inch until you have a new head of healthy hair. The recovery process is frustrating and many women just dive in and cut it all off and start over with a flattering short and sassy look. Either way, you have to be patient and know that it will grow back.

Question

I'm recovering from breast cancer and my hair has thinned and shed. I am looking for an inexpensive, easy to care for and conservative (but not matronly) style. What cut and shape will flatter my diamond-shaped face?

Answer

First of all, let me congratulate you on your recovery. Be encouraged by your healing and stay positive. An important part of getting back on track is your appearance. Choosing the right style for your facial shape and your lifestyle is a smart approach. To flatter your diamond-shaped face, go for soft layering and volume at the top crown and neck area. Stay away from styles that add fullness or volume at the ear and cheek area in that this will create more fullness in an area you want to minimize. A great cut that flatters makes style upkeep effortless and easy to maintain.

Question

My hair is very thin, and I don't go to salons because I am ashamed of my hair. Is there any way to grow my hair back? Is there a way to wear a wig so that people won't know it's a wig? I am considering a lace front wig; what are your thoughts?

Answer

If your hair has not always been thin then you may want to see a Hair Restoration Specialist or see your doctor to make sure the thinning is not the result of a health imbalance or genetic predisposition. You really want to understand the cause of your thinning condition and if possible regain some of your hair's fullness. In the meantime, if you are interested in a natural-looking wig, we are living in a time when you have choices. My first suggestion is to choose a wig made of human hair vs synthetic fibers. Human hair will cost more, but will look more natural and can last a very long time, in addition to the fact that you can shampoo, condition, and re-style with as many looks as the length will allow.

Lastly, lace front wigs can now be purchased in beauty stores or online, and can be ordered from your trusted stylists. Look for a professional who specializes in helping individuals with hair thinning and hair loss with private rooms to maintain confidentiality. If you want your wig to fit like it is natural, your proper measurements will need to be provided for custom fit. I recommend that you go to a professional stylist who does this as part of his or her business for proper fit and application.

One word of caution regarding lace front wigs: these wigs were designed with entertainers or hair loss patients in mind. They have now become mainstream, and if the application process and removal is not done properly, the adhesive that is used to hold the wig in place can cause additional hair loss, so proceed with caution.

Question

My hair is uneven, damaged, and will not grow. Can you recommend any products to help make my hair grow?

Answer

I often hear women say that their hair doesn't grow, but your hair is growing an average of one quarter to one half inch a month. Often due to damage, hair may be breaking off as quickly as it grows.

My best suggestion, if your hair is uneven and damaged, is that you take action and get a good haircut to eliminate the damaged hair. Damaged hair will not heal or correct itself, and will continue to split and damage your healthy hair. If you don't get a stylish cut, then your hair will eventually cut itself through breakage.

Next, condition, condition, condition — give your hair the balance of protein and moisture it so desperately needs, in a two-step process. First, use the protein strengthener of your choice to fortify your weak strands; this will enable your hair to withstand future wear and tear. Next, use the moisturizing conditioner of your choice to soften, moisturize, and restore flexibility to your hair. This creates a pattern for future hair health. To keep it looking great, trim every 8 weeks, and use regular conditioning balancing protein and moisture, and your bad hair days will be over.

Question

I have multi-ethnic hair that is naturally curly and wavy. I flat iron my hair often and have split ends? What can I do?

Answer

If your ends are split, a good trim is in order. Your hair strand is held together by glue — like and spring-like proteins; every time you use heat on your hair the proteins soften a little to allow your hair to take the shape of your heat implement (flatiron, curling iron, crimping iron…). Too much heat, along with daily wear and tear, blow drying, combing, brushing, and rubber band pony tail holders, cause the adhesives that hold the hair fiber together to be lost and the hair strand unravels, like thread — we call it a split end. You can use conditioning products to hold the splits together temporarily, but the best cure is to trim away the split so it cannot continue to split up the strand and damage the new healthy hair. Reduce your use of heat. Find a low-maintenance style you don't have to curl or flatiron every day. Condition to fortify your weak strands with a balance of protein and moisture, and in no time you will love your hair again.

Question

My hair continuously falls out; it falls out even more when I'm stressed. My hair is also dry and feels rough to the touch. What kind of products will help the condition of my hair to improve?

Answer

Is your hair breaking off, or is it falling out? The difference is that hair breakage is external, and is likely caused by some of your hair-styling habits. Hair loss is internal and is likely caused by stress, hormonal imbalance, medication, or genetic pre-disposition. Your approach to a solution will depend on the cause. Start with a nutritional supplement to build you up and nourish your hair growth system. Look for ingredients like biotin, B5, zinc, and amino acids. These ingredients will pump up your hair follicle's metabolism and promote growth. It takes the cells around your follicles about 90 days to rejuvenate, so be patient, and in about 3 months the internal contributors will be restored and a better quality of hair will begin growing in.

You should also get a good physical to be certain that all is well with your health. Excessive hair loss can be the sign of some type of deficiency, hormonal or health issue. Once you know the cause of your hair loss, it will be easier to address your particular needs.

Question
I got my hair cut because I thought that it would promote hair growth. However, I have noticed that the top of my hair is breaking off and one side of my hair is thicker than the rest. What can I do to make my hair thick all over and make the top grow back?

Answer
Haircuts remove the split and or damaged ends and allow you to rock a cute new hairstyle. The breakage in the top and sides may have happened separately, but certainly should be addressed. You should deep condition your hair using a balance of protein and moisture-based conditioners. In terms of thickness, that sounds like you may be experiencing some thinning, which may be still a separate issue. Look for nutritional supplements targeted toward promoting hair growth, stimulating hair growth from the inside. The layered approach to hair care will provide benefits inside and out, strengthening existing hair and promoting future hair growth.

Question
Should I shampoo my hair before a relaxer? I am taking out a sew-in weave that I've been wearing for about two months. I have really thick (not coarse) hair and haven't had a perm since two weeks before I got my sew-in weave.

Answer
I'm glad you're asking this question — many weave or extension wearers are not sure how to proceed when coming out of their extensions. When coming out of a weave it is wise to always shampoo and

deep condition at least once, allowing 1 to 2 weeks to pass before getting any chemical service. This time will allow hair to recover from the tension and stress of the weave, and the conditioning step is to revitalize hair that has not had the benefit of proper conditioning during the eight weeks you wore the weave.

Every Strand Matters!

TO LEARN MORE, visit:
www.HairTraumaCenter.com
www.StyleInfinityHTC.com
www.HealthyHairRehabNow.com

TO BOOK JACQUELINE as a speaker, please contact:
Jacqueline Tarrant
Style Infinity
Hair Trauma Center
155 N Michigan Ave – Suite 606
Chicago, IL 60601
(312) 529-7043
Email: HairTraumaDr@gmail.com

www.ingramcontent.com/pod-product-compliance
Lightning Source LLC
Chambersburg PA
CBHW060627290526
45793CB00001B/171